and Management of

Skin and Soft-Tissue Infections®

Thomas M. File, Jr., MS, MD

Chief, Infectious Disease Service
Summa Health System
Akron, Ohio
Professor of Internal Medicine
Head, Infectious Disease Section
Northeastern Ohio Universities College of Medicine
Rootstown, Ohio

Dennis L. Stevens, MD, PhD

Chief, Infectious Disease Section
Veterans Affairs Medical Center
Boise, Idaho
Professor of Medicine
University of Washington School of Medicine,
Seattle

Second Edition

Published by Handbooks in Health Care Co.,
Newtown, Pennsylvania, USA

International Standard Book Number: 978-1-884065-77-4

Library of Congress Catalog Card Number: 2007935622

Table of Contents

This book has been prepared and is presented as a service to the medical community. The information provided reflects the knowledge, experience, and personal opinions of Thomas M. File, Jr., MS, MD, Chief, Infectious Disease Service, Summa Health System, Akron, Ohio, and Professor of Internal Medicine and Head, Infectious Disease Section, Northeastern Ohio Universities College of Medicine, Rootstown, Ohio, and Dennis L. Stevens, MD, PhD, Chief, Infectious Disease Section, Veterans Affairs Medical Center, Boise, Idaho, and Professor of Medicine, University of Washington School of Medicine, Seattle.

This book is not intended to replace or to be used as a substitute for the complete prescribing information prepared by each manufacturer for each drug. Because of possible variations in drug indications, in dosage information, in newly described toxicities, in drug/drug interactions, and in other items of importance, reference to such complete prescribing information is definitely recommended before any of the drugs discussed are used or prescribed.

Dedications

Dr. File wishes to dedicate this book to his mother, Ruth; his late father, Thomas; his wife, Mary; and his children, Elizabeth and Jason.

Dr. Stevens wishes to dedicate this book to his mother, Alma; his late father, John; his wife, Amy; and his children, Karsten (deceased) and Marisa.

Chapter **1**

Introduction

nfections of the skin and soft tissue are among the most common disorders treated by primary care physicians. These infections range from mild pyodermas to life-threatening necrotizing infections. The skin provides the initial major barrier between humans and their environment. Consequently, manifestations of skin infections are easily detected because patients readily recognize inflammatory changes on their skin.

Skin and soft-tissue infections are treated by all medical branches, but particularly by primary care physicians, surgeons, and dermatologists. According to information obtained from 1980 through 1996 from national databases maintained by the Centers for Disease Control and Prevention's National Center for Health Statistics (NCHS), skin infections represent the fourth most common infection that results in outpatient visits in the United States. The top three are respiratory tract infections; upper respiratory tract infections, such as sinusitis and otitis media and externa; and lower respiratory tract infections, such as influenza. The overall rate of outpatient visits for skin infections was 48.3/1,000 population. In a similar database, cellulitis was a common cause for admission to hospitals, with a rate of 129/100,000 population. The United States Agency for Health Care Policy and Research ranked cellulitis as the 28th most common diagnosis in hospitalized patients in 1996; and one review cited statistics that cellulitis accounted for 2.2% of office visits among 320,000 members of a health-care plan in Utah in 1999.

The skin is exposed to many potential insults, including any form of surgery and injuries that disrupt skin continuity. In addition, local or systemic diseases can interrupt skin integrity, such as local trauma, pressure ulcers, and disorders that impair arterial or venous blood flow. A break in the integrity of the epidermis or deeper layers of the soft tissue allows micro-organisms that are typically nonpathogenic colonizers of normal skin to become pathogenic.

A myriad of microbes may cause skin and soft tissue infections, but the most common pathogens are *Staphylococcus aureus* (*S aureus*) and *Streptococcus pyogenes* (*S pyogenes*). Community-acquired methicillin-resistant *S aureus* (CA-MRSA) has emerged as a significant and common cause of community skin infections over the past several years and has changed the approach to empirical management of community-acquired skin infections. The emergence of CA-MRSA has increased the importance of obtaining cultures of even mild skin infections. Infections of the skin and soft tissue can be classified as primary pyodermas, secondary infections associated with underlying conditions of the skin, and necrotizing infections.

Primary pyodermas are skin infections that usually originate in healthy skin and occur in the absence of underlying conditions. These pyodermas are usually caused by a single organism. Secondary infections develop in association with pre-existing lesions (ie, surgical or traumatic wounds, ulcers) that serve as portals for the entry of pathogens. Secondary infections are frequently polymicrobial. Necrotizing infections are also often found in association with underlying conditions. They are commonly life threatening and require expeditious recognition and intervention for optimal patient outcome. We have organized this handbook according to these classifications.

Chapter **2**

Pathophysiology

B acterial skin infections range from mild pyodermas to life-threatening necrotizing infections. The likelihood of a skin or soft-tissue infection occurring depends on several factors: the number and virulence of the microorganism, the tropism of the pathogen, and the presence of several host factors. The manifestations of bacterial skin infections result from the interaction of bacterial virulence factors with the immune status and underlying conditions of the host (Table 2-1).

Anatomy

Knowledge of the anatomy of the skin and soft tissues is important to understand the pathophysiology of infections to these structures. The skin is composed of several layers: the epidermis, the dermis, subcutaneous fat, fascia, and muscle (Figure 2-1). The epidermis is an avascular sheet of constantly renewing cells that covers the entire body. The basal layer of the epidermis is composed of keratinocytes, which divide, differentiate, and are eventually sloughed from the surface. As they rise from the basal layer to the surface, they become more stratified, producing a tough layer of dead cells, the stratum corium. The stratum corium becomes a protective sheath that provides both an important permeability barrier and a wall that excludes most environmental pathogens.

In addition to the keratinocytes, the epidermis contains other cell types, the Langerhans' cells and the pigment-containing melanocytes. Langerhans' cells are fixed-tissue macrophages. They represent a portion of the immune system and process antigens that may breach the stratum corium.

Table 2-1: Microbe and Host Factors That Affect Bacterial Skin Infections

Bacterial Virulence Factors

- Adherence factors (ie, fibrils on M-protein of *S pyogenes*)
- Antiphagocytic factors (ie, M-protein, C5A peptidase of *S pyogenes*)
- Enzymes (proteinases, hyaluronidases, phospholipases)
- Toxins (ie, toxic shock syndrome [TSS] toxin, exfoliatin)
- β-lactamase production (reduces susceptibility to β-lactam antibiotics)
- Panton-Valentine leukocidin (PVL) cytotoxin

Local Defense Factors

- Intact skin (barrier effect)
- Low hydrogen ion concentration (pH)
- Relative dryness
- Antibacterial secretions of sebaceous glands

Host Conditions

- Abnormalities of epidermis (eczema, dermatitis)
- Breaks of skin (abrasions; trauma; insect, human, and animal bites; surgical incision)
- Ulcers (diabetic foot pressure sores)
- Ischemia
- Immunosuppression
- Presence of foreign body (ie, catheter, slivers)

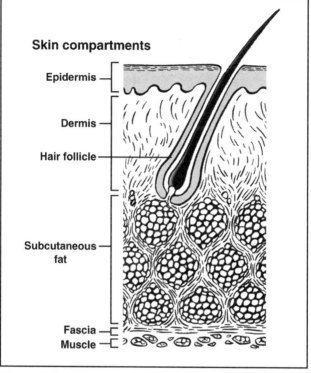

Skin compartments

- Epidermis
- Dermis
- Hair follicle
- Subcutaneous fat
- Fascia
- Muscle

Figure 2-1: Anatomy of the skin and the underlying layers of soft tissue. From: Gorbach SL, Bartlett JG, Blacklow NR: *Infectious Diseases,* 3rd ed. Philadelphia, PA, Lippincott Williams & Wilkins, p 1151. Used with permission.

The thickness of the epidermis is, on average, 0.1 mm, but may reach 0.8 mm on the palms and 1.4 mm on the soles.

The dermis is several millimeters thick and is separated from the epidermis by a basement membrane. Within the dermis are collagen and elastin, which are embedded within a glycoprotein matrix; these provide strength and resilience to the skin. Blood vessels, lymphatics, and fibroblasts are also located within the dermis, as are skin appendages, eccrine sweat glands, sebaceous glands, and hair follicles. All of these may be involved in infections. These appendages may contain organisms of the normal skin flora, but they are also susceptible to invasion by pathogens because they are associated with gaps in the stratum corium.

The thickness of subcutaneous fat varies over the body. It consists principally of lipid cells and provides an effective cushion for the skin. Beneath the subcutaneous fat, the superficial fascia separates the skin from underlying muscle and may provide a pathway for the spread of infection from micro-organisms.

The Relationship of the Skin and Micro-organisms

The skin represents an effective physical barrier against invasion from micro-organisms. Normal skin of healthy individuals is resistant to invasion by bacteria that may reside innocuously on the surface. Skin infection usually occurs when there is a defect in the integrity of the epidermis, allowing micro-organisms that have colonized the skin to invade the tissue and cause clinical manifestations. Such defects can result from surgery, from trauma, or from relatively innocuous insults, such as an insect bite or an abrasion. Skin lesions can also be caused by hematogenous spread from distal infections by bacteria or bacterial toxins.

Most bacteria will decrease in number when applied to the surface of the keratinized layers of normal skin. Furthermore, these physical characteristics of skin act to reduce bacterial multiplication:
- the relatively low pH (approximately 5.5) of the skin environment;
- the presence of natural antibacterial substances in the secretions of the sebaceous glands;
- the relative dryness of normal skin;
- bacterial interference, which is the suppressive effect of normal flora on the growth of pathogens.

Normal skin is colonized with a variety of micro-organisms that are classified as resident flora. These organisms include *Propionibacterium* species, coagulase-negative staphylococci, and *Corynebacterium* species. For the most part, these organisms are not pathogenic. When a foreign body, such as an intravenous catheter, is introduced, these resident organisms may cause localized infection and bacteremia. *Staphylococcus aureus* and β-hemolytic streptococci, which are more likely to cause invasive disease, may transiently colonize the skin. In addition, members of the Enterobacteriaceae family, *Pseudomonas* species, *Enterococcus* species, and a variety of anaerobes are particularly prone to colonizing the lower extremities (derived from fecal sources). Colonization of normal skin with pathogenic organisms usually precedes clinical infection. Subsequently, even minimal trauma may cause an epidermal defect that allows skin organisms to cross the keratinized layers that normally would protect against infection and, thus, cause disease. Although the causative pathogens associated with many of the pyodermas are fairly predictable (usually *S aureus* or β-hemolytic *Streptococcus* species) other organisms may be involved (eg, *Pseudomonas* in whirlpool folliculitis, anaerobes and *Enterobacteriaceae* in chronic hidradenitis suppurativa, and *Pasteurella multocida* in animal bites).

S aureus frequently colonizes both outpatients and hospitalized patients. Common sites for colonization include the anterior nares or perineum. Approximately 50% of patients carry *S aureus* transiently at any given time. Individuals who are prone to colonization include health-care workers, diabetic patients, patients receiving chronic hemodialysis, and users of illicit intravenous drugs. Most patients with staphylococcal folliculitis or furunculosis experience a self-limiting infection. Certain patients, however, are especially prone to recurrent infections, including those who have (1) hypogammaglobulinemia, (2) diabetes mellitus, (3) cancer or have undergone organ transplants and are receiving immunosuppressant drugs,

(4) chronic granulomatous disease of childhood, or (5) Job syndrome. In addition, poor hygiene, obesity, folliculosis, chronic dermatitis, seborrhea, psoriasis, malnutrition, and occupational trauma may predispose the patient to recurrent *S aureus* pyoderma.

Virulence Factors

The pathogenicity of specific micro-organisms is determined in part by virulence factors. Local invasiveness is an important element in group A streptococcal infection (*Streptococcus pyogenes*), which depends on the antiphagocytic M-protein of the bacterial cell envelope. Several extracellular products associated with *S pyogenes* may contribute to the manifestations of skin infection. These include hyaluronidase, proteinase, DNAse, and streptokinase, all of which cause liquefaction of pus and enhance spread throughout tissue planes. Toxins and enzymes appear to play a role in the ability of *S aureus* to produce disease. α and δ toxins may contribute to disease manifestations by damaging tissue membranes. Exfoliative toxin, which is produced by certain strains of *S aureus*, causes separation of the epidermis from the dermis, resulting in the scalded skin syndrome.

Both *S aureus* and *S pyogenes* may produce pyrogenic toxins associated with a toxic shock syndrome (TSS). The staphylococcal TSS characterized by hypotension, rash, and multisystem involvement is caused by strains of *S aureus* that produce an exotoxin, TSS toxin-1 (TSST-1). The occurrence of serious skin infections that result from *S pyogenes* and are characterized by necrotizing fasciitis has been described and defined as group A *Streptococcus* (GAS) TSS (see Chapter 8). More recently, community-acquired methicillin-resistant *S aureus* (CA-MRSA) strains are recognized as common cause of skin infections, and can be associated with necrotizing manifestations (discussed in detail in Chapter 3). The potential of CA-MRSA strains to cause serious illness is further emphasized by their production of a relatively greater number of recognized staphylococcal virulence factors when compared with other strains of *S aureus*. Most notably, CA-MRSA strains frequently carry the Panton-Valentine leukocidin (PVL) genes, which produce cytotoxins associated with tissue necrosis and leukocyte destruction.

The pathogenesis of skin infections associated with gram-negative bacilli (eg, exotoxins produced by *Pseudomonas aeruginosa*) and anaerobes may be due to elaboration of a variety of extracellular toxins. In the case of *Clostridium perfringens*, elaboration of collagenases, specific toxins, and proteases appear to play important roles in producing the spreading necrotizing infection that may be associated with this organism.

Host Response

Once organisms penetrate the barrier of the epidermis and dermis, either through defects (eg, abrasions) or through natural gaps (eg, hair follicles), a rich plexus of capillaries beneath the dermis delivers the components of the host's defenses (including oxygen, complement, immunoglobulin, macrophages, lymphocytes, and granulocytes) to the site of infection. Virtually all bacteria are composed of specific proteins, which are chemoattractive to phagocytic cells (ie, granulocytes, macrophages). Microbial cell wall components such as endotoxins of gram-negative bacteria and peptidoglycan of gram-positive bacteria activate the alternative complement pathway, yielding serum-derived chemotactic factors. Polymorphonuclear leukocytes leave the capillaries through efflux through endothelial cell junctions and follow the gradient of chemotactic factors derived from the bacteria and serum to the site of infection. Involved endothelial cells also produce chemotactic cytokines, such as interleukin-8 (IL-8), which also serves as a potent chemoattractant for leukocytes. Production of proinflammatory cytokines (eg, interleukin-1 [IL-1], tumor necrosis factor-α [TNF-α], and interleukin-6 [IL-6]) occurs after the initiation of infection and augments the host immune functions. These cytokines induce fever, activate neutrophils, and increase antibody production and the synthesis of acute phase reactants, such as C-reactive protein (CRP). Cytokine-driven stimulation of endothelial cells results in vasodilation. The net effect is greater blood flow to the skin and soft tissues. These processes result in the cardinal manifestations of inflammation: heat, swelling, erythema, and pain.

Host Factors

Several host factors contribute to the predisposition for skin infections: reduced vascular supply, compromised immune system, disruption of lymphatic or venous drainage, and the presence of underlying conditions, such as dermatitis or a foreign body (intravenous catheter or suture).

Skin infections more commonly occur in warm, humid conditions. Poverty, crowding, close contact (eg, between classmates, athletes, and soldiers), and poor personal hygiene promote impetigo, which is easily spread within families and other closely associated groups of people. Infection typically arises at the site of minor skin trauma such as insect bites or abrasions.

Decreased blood flow, which may occur from factors such as pressure, thrombosis, or drugs predispose skin to infection. Compounds such as corticosteroids, which inhibit phospholipase A_2 activity, and nonsteroidal anti-inflammatory agents, which inhibit cyclo-oxygenase, reduce local blood flow to tissues. Thus, these agents are often used in inflammatory conditions because they reduce pain and swelling. However, if the inflammation is due to bacterial infection, these drugs may predispose the patient to more severe infection or mask the clinical signs and delay the diagnosis of skin infection. Other conditions that may reduce tissue perfusion include peripheral vascular disease (PVD); diabetes mellitus with microvascular disease; chronic venous stasis causing capillary obstruction; and pressure necrosis.

Polymicrobial (Aerobic/Anaerobic) Infections

There are numerous examples of mixed bacterial infections in clinical medicine. The polymicrobial nature of peritonitis and intra-abdominal abscess formation is well known. In skin and soft-tissue infections, a polymicrobial etiology can often be found with surgical site infections, bite wound infections, pressure ulcer infections, and diabetic foot infections. A mixture of anaerobic and aerobic organisms found in such infections may act to produce a synergistic infection. Synergy is the cooperative interaction of two or more bacterial species that produces a clinical infection usually more severe than one achieved by an individual bacterial species acting alone. Gram-positive organisms such as *Staphylococcus* and *Streptococcus*, gram-negative enteric bacilli, and anaerobes are frequently isolated from these infections. In combination, these organisms may induce the formation of abscesses and often result in severe necrotizing infections. The pathogenic role of mixed flora is examined in greater detail in Chapters 6 and 7.

Selected Readings

Bisno AL, Stevens DL: Streptococcal infections of skin and soft tissues. *N Engl J Med* 1996;334:240-245.

Brook I, Frazier EH: Clinical features and aerobic and anaerobic characteristics of cellulitis. *Arch Surg* 1995;130:786-792.

File TM Jr: Skin Infections. In: Tan JS, ed: *Expert Guide to Infectious Diseases*. Philadelphia, PA, American College of Physicians, 2002, pp 605-617.

File TM Jr, Tan JS: Treatment of bacterial skin and soft tissue infections. *Surg Gynecol Obstet* 1991;S172:17-24.

Finch R: Skin and soft tissues infections. *Lancet* 1988;1:164-168.

Schluter B, Konig W: Microbial pathogenicity and host defense mechanisms: crucial parameters of posttraumatic infections. *Thorac Cardiovasc Surg* 1990;38:339-347.

Stevens DL, Bisno AL, Chambers HF, et al, and the Infectious Diseases Society of America: Practice guidelines for the diagnosis and management of skin and soft-tissue infections. *Clin Infect Dis* 2005;41:1373-1406.

Stevens DL: Cellulitis, pyoderma, abscesses and other skin and subcutaneous infections. In: Cohen J, Powderly WG, et al (eds): *Infectious Diseases,* 2nd ed. Edinburgh, Scotland, Mosby, 2003, pp 133-144.

Swartz MN and Pasternack MS: Cellulitis and subcutaneous tissue infections. In: Mandell GL, Bennett JE, Dolin R, eds: *Principles and Practice of Infectious Diseases*, 6th ed. New York, NY, Elsevier Science, 2005, pp 1172-1193.

Chapter **3**

Methicillin-resistant *Staphylococcus aureus* (MRSA) Infections

S ince its first appearance in 1970, methicillin-resistant *Staphylococcus aureus* (*S aureus*) (MRSA) has been a growing problem. These organisms are resistant to all β-lactam antibiotics because of a penicillin-binding protein (PBP) with a low affinity for β-lactam antibiotics (ie, PBP-2A). In the mid-1970s, the infection appeared as a hospital-acquired MRSA (HA-MRSA) and has increased dramatically in most large hospitals over the past 30 years (Figure 3-1). Although hospitals are still the most common settings for MRSA, the organisms have also become a serious problem in long-term care facilities and are increasingly being recognized in communities at large (community-acquired [CA]-MRSA).

Genetic and Phenotypic Differences in CA-MRSA and HA-MRSA Infections

Epidemiologic and molecular studies have determined that CA-MRSA and HA-MRSA strains are extremely different. Daum and colleagues have demonstrated that a chromosomal cassette containing the mecA gene is much larger in HA-MRSA strains than in CA-MRSA strains. In fact, there are at least three different mec cassettes (ie, that harbor the mecA gene) in HA-MRSA strains (mec cassette types I, II, and III) and one in CA-MRSA strains (mec cassette type IV). The larger types I, II, and III cassettes also

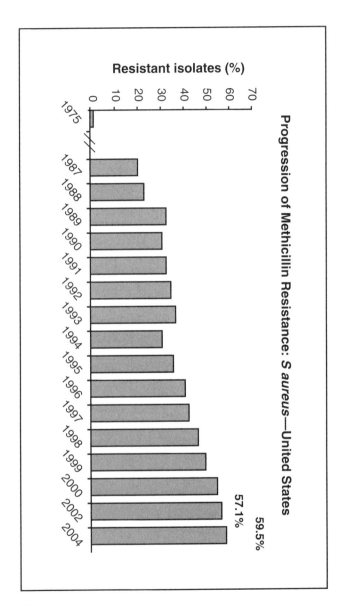

Resistant isolates (%)

Progression of Methicillin Resistance: *S aureus*—United States

2004
2002 — 59.5%
2000 — 57.1%
1999
1998
1997
1996
1995
1994
1993
1992
1991
1990
1989
1988
1987
1975

carry genetic determinants for antibiotic resistance. As a result, HA-MRSA strains tend to be more resistant to a variety of antibiotics, such as erythromycin, clindamycin (Cleocin HCl®), tetracycline, gentamicin, and the fluoroquinolones than CA-MRSA strains.

CA-MRSA strains carry more toxin genes than HA-MRSA strains, and this may partially explain the ability of CA-MRSA strains to cause novel and more aggressive infections. For example, CA-MRSA strains have been associated with necrotizing fasciitis, pyomyositis, Fredrickson-Waterhouse syndrome, toxic shock syndrome (TSS), and hemorrhagic necrotizing pneumonitis following influenza infection. Recent studies suggest that a high percentage of MRSA strains possess TSS toxin-1 (TSST-1), staphylococcal enterotoxins, and Panton-Valentine leukocidin (PVL) cytotoxin. PVL cytotoxin has been found in 75% of CA-MRSA strains and in 100% of strains isolated from patients with necrotizing fasciitis, necrotizing pneumonitis, and pyomyositis. It is a two-component exotoxin that assembles on the surface of neutrophils. The role of PVL cytotoxin in human infections is unproven, although there have been experimental studies that have clearly demonstrated that the cytotoxin is an important virulence factor in animal models of pneumonia.

Figure 3-1: Increase in prevalence of MRSA among hospital isolates in the United States over time. Examination of the rates of methicillin-resistant *Staphylococcus aureus* (MRSA) isolates in the United States by the Centers for Disease Control and Prevention (CDC) shows that MRSA rates have increased steadily over the past decade, with a dramatic 40% increase over the past 5-year historical mean. In 2000, 55.3% of the *S aureus* isolates associated with a hospital-acquired infection in intensive care unit (ICU) patients were resistant to methicillin, reflecting a further 31% increase in resistant *S aureus* isolates in 2001.

Empiric Treatment
of Staphylococcal Infections

The empiric treatment of staphylococcal infections has become complex due to the rapid increase in the prevalence of both CA-MRSA and HA-MRSA. The decision to select a given antibiotic and its route of administration must be based upon the seriousness of the infection, the trends in staphylococcal resistance patterns (ie, percentage of strains that are MRSA) in the specific geographic area, and the established risk factors for MRSA infection in a given patient.

Treatment of Minor Staphylococcal Infections

Minor staphylococcal infections of the skin, such as folliculitis, furunculosis, paronychia, and styes, generally respond well to the topical application of warm soaks. Larger focal infections, such as carbuncles or deep abscesses, frequently require incision and drainage. Concomitant antibiotic treatment is indicated in the following situations:

1. When the infection is associated with systemic signs of infection, ie, fever or tachycardia
2. When lesions are large, numerous, or recurrent
3. When surgical drainage alone has failed
4. If patients have underlying medical problems, ie, valvular heart disease or implanted prosthetic devices
5. When the nose or face is involved.

Cloxacillin (Cloxapen®) or dicloxacillin (Dynapen®) in an oral dosage of 250 to 500 mg every 6 hours is generally sufficient for methicillin-susceptible *S aureus* (MSSA). Alternatives would be an oral cephalosporin, erythromycin, clindamycin, or the newer macrolides (see Chapter 4).

Treatment of Major Staphylococcal Infections With No Risk Factors for MRSA

For serious staphylococcal skin infections, such as cellulitis, deep-wound sepsis, or necrotizing fasciitis, parenteral antibiotics are mandatory. Oxacillin (Bactocill®) or nafcillin in a dosage of 1 to 2 g every 4 hours or a parenteral cephalosporin, such as cephalothin, cefuroxime axetil (Ceftin®), or cefuroxime sodium (Zinacef®), are excellent alternatives. Constitutive resistance to erythromycin is common among HA-MRSA strains and in certain geographic regions. Inducible clindamycin resistance is increasing in prevalence in both CA-MRSA and HA-MRSA strains. In addition, the usage of ciprofloxacin (Cipro®, ProQuin® XR) and even the new quinolones is limited by the emergence of resistance. Interestingly, trimethoprim/sulfamethoxazole (TMP/SMX) (Bactrim™, Septra®) remains active against both methicillin-susceptible *S aureus* (MSSA) and MRSA strains. Anecdotally, TMP/SMX also is commonly used to treat MRSA complicated skin and skin-structure infections (cSSSIs), although there are few, if any, data showing its efficacy in comparative trials.

Serious Staphylococcal Infections With a High Likelihood of MRSA

Empiric treatment of severe staphylococcal soft-tissue infections should be with an agent that has proven efficacy against MRSA at least until antibiotic susceptibilities are available. Vancomycin has been the workhorse antibiotic to treat all MRSA infections; however, numerous problems have emerged. With the increased use of vancomycin, strains of *S aureus* have appeared that are resistant to vancomycin with minimum inhibitory concentrations (MICs) of >16 µg/mL (vancomycin-resistant *S aureus* [VRSA]). Although these organisms are uncommon in the United States, vigorous control measures are required to prevent them from joining vancomycin-resistant enterococci (VRE) as major nosocomial pathogens. Vancomycin-intermediate MRSA (VISA) with MICs of 2 to 4 µg/mL and heteroresistant strains with MICs of 4 to 16 µg/mL have also appeared. Heteroresistance can only be detected in broth culture in the presence of a very large inocula (10^7

colony-forming units [CFUs]/mL). There also is mounting evidence that over the course of three to four decades of vancomycin usage, MICs have gradually increased, even in sensitive strains. This development has relevance to the treatment of skin and soft-tissue infections because tissue penetration of vancomycin may only reach 2 to 4 μg/mL. In the past, MRSA strains commonly had MICs of 0.1 to 0.5 μg/mL, values considerably below achievable tissue levels of vancomycin (Vancocin®), which was sufficient. As suggested, at the present time and in the future, we may encounter strains with MICs of 1 to 2 μg/mL, which may account for the greater failure rate of vancomycin in the treament of a variety of infections including those involving the skin and soft tissue.

New Antibiotics to Treat MRSA Infections

Linezolid (Zyvox®), daptomycin (Cubicin®), quinupristin/dalfopristin (Synercid®), tigecycline (Tygacil®), and antibiotics currently not available in the United States—ceftobiprole, iclaprim, teicoplanin, and telavancin—are newer antibiotics with activity against MRSA (Table 3-1).

Teicoplanin, a glycopeptide antimicrobial, is approved for the treatment of staphylococcal cSSSIs in Europe, but not in the United States.

Daptomycin and tigecycline have been approved for skin and soft-tissue infections, including MRSA, in the United States. Daptomycin's mechanism of action involves the formation of pores in the cell membranes of bacteria with rapid loss of intracellular potassium (Table 3-2).

Tigecycline, a minocycline derivative that inhibits protein synthesis, has been approved for cSSSIs in the United States (Table 3-2). Linezolid also inhibits protein synthesis (Table 3-2), but, unlike the other antibiotics in this class, it prevents the initiation of the formation of the complex of transfer ribonucleic acid (tRNA), messenger ribonucleic acid (mRNA), and ribosome. As a result, cross-resistance to other types of protein synthesis inhib-

Table 3-1: New Antibiotics With Activity Against MRSA

Antibiotic	FDA Status
Vancomycin	FDA approved
Linezolid (Zyvox®)	FDA approved
Daptomycin (Cubicin®)	FDA approved
Tigecycline (Tygacil®)	FDA approved
Dalbavancin	FDA letter
Iclaprim	Phase III clinical trials
Ceftobiprole	Phase III clinical trials
Telavancin	Phase III clinical trials

FDA=US Food and Drug Administration

itors is not possible. Linezolid has been approved in the United States for skin and soft-tissue infections as well as nosocomial and community-acquired pneumonias (CAPs) caused by MRSA, and evidence is accumulating that, like clindamycin, linezolid is a potent suppressor of toxin production by staphylococcus strains. Because of this characteristic, linezolid may be a more suitable agent to use in patients with staphylococcal TSS or necrotizing fasciitis caused by PVL-producing strains. In vitro, daptomycin and linezolid have shown excellent activity against VISA and VRSA.

Taking quinupristin/dalfopristin has led to a high incidence of phlebitis and myopathy. As a result, its use requires a central line placement. Dalbavancin and telavancin are also glycopeptide antibiotics that effect cell wall synthesis by interfering with cross-linking. In addition, telavancin affects the integrity of bacterial cell membranes (Table

Table 3-2: Mechanisms of Action of New Antibiotics With Activity Against MRSA

Antibiotic	Mechanism of Action
Vancomycin	Cell wall
Daptomycin	Cell membrane
Linezolid	Protein synthesis
Dalbavancin*	Cell wall
Quinupristin/ dalfopristin (Synercid®)	Protein synthesis
Tigecycline	Protein synthesis
Telavancin*	Cell wall and cell membrane
Iclaprim*	Folic acid inhibition
Ceftobiprole*	PBP and cell wall

PBP=penicillin-binding protein
*Not yet approved for use in the United States.

3-2). Dalbavancin has an extremely long half-life and is given by intravenous (IV) injection of 1-g dose and, 7 days later, 500 mg IV. In clinical trials of cSSSIs, the efficacy of telavancin was noninferior to vancomycin. Iclaprim is a folic acid antagonist with 4- to 10-fold higher activity against staphylococci than TMP/SMX. Ceftobiprole has excellent activity against MRSA isolates, even though it is a cephalosporin. Phase III clinical trials for ceftobiprole and iclaprim have been completed, and the results of those trials are currently being evaluated by the US Food and Drug Administration (FDA).

Prevention and Infection Control Measures

Epidemiologic control of staphylococcal infections requires the ongoing surveillance and reporting of infections. The dramatic increase in the prevalence of MRSA in community and hospital environments is proof of the difficulty of controlling the spread of these microbes. Contact precautions should be followed in the management of patients with active infections of the skin or of wounds. There has been a movement among infection control practitioners to culture the nares of all patients admitted to hospitals in an effort to define patients at risk for MRSA. However, the treatment of these nasal or rectal carriers can be frustrating, particularly if the carriers are hospital personnel or persons suffering from recurrent furunculosis. Topical treatment with germicidal soaps, povidone-iodine solution, or antibiotic ointments has been advocated, but long-term results have been disappointing. Topical mupirocin 2% ointment (Bactroban®, Centany™) can reduce the MRSA carrier rate, but, because recolonization is common, mupirocin is not recommended for extended use in long-term care facilities. Orally administered antibiotics, including rifampin (Rifadin®, Rimactane®), TMP-SMX, and ciprofloxacin, have also failed to live up to initially promising findings. Bacterial interference, which attempts to replace epidemiologically virulent strains of staphylococci with strains that have been deliberately colonized to be less virulent, has generally been abandoned, in part because infections have been caused by these supposedly less virulent strains. Attempts to develop staphylococcal vaccines are continuing. In a recent clinical trial in dialysis patients, a staphylococcal surface carbohydrate conjugated to *Pseudomonas* exotoxin A significantly reduced the incidence of bacteremia, although the protective antibodies lasted only 8 months.

A placebo-controlled trial of nasal mupirocin (Bactroban®) in 34 patients who were *S aureus* carriers found that a monthly course of nasal mupirocin reduced the incidence of nasal colonization and skin infections for at least 1 year.

However, because resistance to mupirocin and recolonization after therapy can occur, indiscriminate use of mupirocin should be avoided.

Summary

The MRSA epidemic has evolved rapidly, and new data are needed regarding the efficacy of older agents, such as tetracycline, clindamycin, and TMP/SMX in the treatment of MRSA infections. Because of the high prevalence of MRSA in hospitals and in the community, we are probably at the tipping point where practitioners should select agents with proven clinical trial efficacy for the treatment of MRSA infections. This recommendation can be stated with more confidence in seriously ill patients. As a result, a practitioner can confidently select one of the agents listed in Table 3-1 to treat a seriously ill patient. Because of the increased expense of those agents, it is more important than ever to make a correct microbial diagnosis and obtain antibiotic susceptibilities. It may then be possible to step down to an older, and cheaper, antibiotic to complete the course of therapy.

Selected Readings

Arbeit RD, Maki D, Tally FP, et al: The safety and efficacy of daptomycin for the treatment of complicated skin and skin-structure infections. *Clin Infect Dis* 2004;38:1673-1681.

Bogdanovich T, Ednie LM, Shapiro S, et al: Antistaphylococcal activity of ceftobiprole, a new broad-spectrum cephalosporin. *Antimicrob Agents Chemother* 2005;49:4210-4219.

Breedt J, Teras J, Gardovskis J, et al: Safety and efficacy of tigecycline in treatment of skin and skin structure infections: results of a double-blind phase 3 comparison study with vancomycin-aztreonam. *Antimicrob Agents Chemother* 2005;49:4658-4666.

Daum RS, Ito T, Hiramatsu K, et al: A novel methicillin-resistance cassette in community-acquired methicillin-resistant Staphylococcus aureus isolates of diverse genetic backgrounds. *J Infect Dis* 2002;186:1344-1347.

Ellis-Grosse EJ, Babinchak T, Dartois N, et al, and Tigecycline 300 cSSSI Study Group, Tigecycline 305 cSSSI Study Group: The efficacy and safety of tigecycline in the treatment of skin and skin-structure infections: results of 2 double-blind phase 3 comparison studies with vancomycin-aztreonam. *Clin Infect Dis* 2005;41(suppl 5): S341-S353.

Fowler VG, Jr, Boucher HW, Corey GR, et al, and S. aureus Endocarditis and Bacteremia Study Group: Daptomycin versus standard therapy for bacteremia and endocarditis caused by Staphylococcus aureus. *N Engl J Med* 2006;355:653-665.

Gillet Y, Issartel B, Vanhems P, et al: Association between Staphylococcus aureus strains carrying gene for Panton-Valentine leukocidin and highly lethal necrotising pneumonia in young immunocompetent patients. *Lancet* 2002;359:753-759.

Jauregui LE, Babazadeh S, Seltzer E, et al: Randomized, double-blind comparison of once-weekly dalbavancin versus twice-daily linezolid therapy for the treatment of complicated skin and skin structure infections. *Clin Infect Dis* 2005;41:1407-1415.

Miller LG, Perdreau-Remington F, Rieg G, et al: Necrotizing fasciitis caused by community-associated methicillin-resistant Staphylococcus aureus in Los Angeles. *N Engl J Med* 2005;352:1445-1453.

Moran GJ, Krishnadasan A, Gorwitz RJ, et al, and EMERGEncy ID Net Study Group: Methicillin-resistant S. aureus infections among patients in the emergency department. *N Engl J Med* 2006;355: 666-674.

Stevens DL, Herr D, Lampiris H, et al: Linezolid versus vancomycin for the treatment of methicillin-resistant Staphylococcus aureus infections. *Clin Infect Dis* 2002;34:1481-1490.

Stevens DL, Smith LG, Bruss JB, et al: Randomized comparison of linezolid (PNU-100766) versus oxacillin-dicloxacillin for treatment of complicated skin and soft tissue infections. *Antimicrob Agents Chemother* 2000;44:3408-3413.

Stryjewski ME, Chu VH, O'Riordan WD, et al, and FAST 2 Investigator Group: Telavancin versus standard therapy for treatment of complicated skin and skin structure infections caused by gram-positive bacteria: FAST 2 study. *Antimicrob Agents Chemother* 2006;50:862-867.

Weigelt J, Itani K, Stevens D, et al, and Linezolid CSSTI Study Group: Linezolid versus vancomycin in treatment of complicated skin and soft tissue infections. *Antimicrob Agents Chemother* 2005;49:2260-2266.

3

Chapter 4

Pyodermas: Superficial Bacterial Skin Infections

Primary superficial skin infections, or pyodermas, usually occur on relatively normal skin in patients who do not exhibit any significant underlying condition. Pyodermas are most often caused by β-hemolytic streptococci, most commonly group A *Streptococcus* (GAS) or *Staphylococcus aureus (S aureus)* (Table 4-1). These infections are often mild, and most do not require parenteral antibiotics or hospitalization. Colonization of normal skin with *Streptococcus pyogenes* or *S aureus* usually precedes clinical infection. Subsequently, minimal trauma—such as may occur with insect bites, scratching, or mild abrasions—may cause enough of an epidermal defect for these organisms to invade the keratinized layers, which normally protect against infection, and cause disease. The clinical manifestations of infection may depend on the depth of the traumatic event, the number of pathogenic organisms, and the patient's underlying response. Pyodermas include folliculitis, furunculosis, carbunculosis, impetigo, cellulitis, erysipelas, and hidradenitis suppurativa.

Streptococcal pyoderma and impetigo occur primarily in children, usually during warm, humid months, when more exposed skin, heat, and moisture cause increased numbers of skin micro-organisms. Predisposing conditions include minor trauma, insect bites, poor hygiene, and pre-existing skin disease (eg, dermatitis).

Folliculitis

Folliculitis is an infection located within hair follicles and the apocrine glands. Folliculitis is most commonly caused by *S aureus*, but gram-negative bacilli or *Candida* species may be the etiologic agents in immunocompromised patients. A specific form of *Pseudomonas* folliculitis has been described in association with whirlpool or hot tub use. An outbreak of pustular dermatitis among mud-wrestling college students also has been described. Organisms isolated from pustules included *Enterobacter cloacae* and *Citrobacter* species. The pathogenesis of this condition may resemble that of pseudomonal folliculitis, with organisms from mud possibly entering the skin through hair follicles or through breaks in the skin caused during wrestling.

Clinically, folliculitis lesions present as 2- to 5-mm erythematous papules that surround a hair follicle and often present with central pustulation (Figure 4-1, see color plate insert). Systemic manifestations are rare. Lesions may spontaneously drain or resolve without scarring. Sycosis barbae is a distinct form of deep folliculitis, often chronic, which occurs on bearded areas.

In whirlpool folliculitis, patients develop generalized, fine, papular pustules from which *Pseudomonas aeruginosa* is commonly isolated (Figure 4-2, see color plate insert). The modified apocrine glands of the external canal of the ear and areola are particularly susceptible to folliculitis. The more common signs and symptoms of this infection include a generalized rash accompanied by otitis externa, mastitis, malaise, and fever. The average incubation period is 2 days. *Pseudomonas* infection commonly follows immersion in swimming pools or hot tubs, where the organism may reside in higher numbers when the chlorination or the pH of the system are not adjusted properly. Whirlpool folliculitis is usually self-limited, although bacteremia has been described. Systemic antibiotics are not indicated unless cellulitis develops or patients are systemically ill.

Table 4-1: Common Microbial Etiology and Antimicrobial Therapy for Superficial Soft-Tissue Infections

Infection	Micro-organisms
Impetigo	*S pyogenes, S aureus* (Almost all bullous impetigo is *S aureus.*)
Cellulitis/ Erysipelas	*S aureus; S pyogenes* (Erysipelas usually *S pyogenes* and other β-hemolytic streptococci)

Therapy and Comments*

Topical: Mupirocin (Bactroban®, Centany™), bacitracin

Oral: Antistaphylococcal penicillin,** first-generation cephalosporin,*** macrolides† (some β-hemolytic streptococci are resistant), clindamycin (300 mg t.i.d.); penicillin VK (250-500 mg b.i.d./q.i.d.) if only group A Streptococcus (GAS) documented

The following if concern for CA-MRSA: Trimethoprim/sulfamethoxazole (TMP/SMX) (1 dose b.i.d., does not cover β-hemolytic streptococci), minocycline (Dynacin®, Minocin®) 100 mg b.i.d., doxycycline (Doryx®, Monodox®, Vibramycin®) 100 mg b.i.d.

Oral: Penicillin VK; if concern for *S aureus*: antistaphylococcal penicillin, first-generation cephalosporin,*** macrolides,† clindamycin (300 mg t.i.d.); levofloxacin (Levaquin®) 500-750 mg q.d., moxifloxacin (Avelox®) 400 mg q.d.

For community-acquired MRSA (CA-MRSA), see impetigo.

IV: Antistaphylococcal penicillin, first-generation cephalosporin,*** clindamycin (600-900 mg q8h);

For MRSA: Vancomycin (15 mg/kg q12h), linezolid (Zyvox®) (600 mg q12h), daptomycin (Cubicin®) (4 mg/kg q24h); tigecycline (Tygacil®) (100 mg initial dose, then 50 mg q12h)

(continued on next page)

Table 4-1: Common Microbial Etiology and Antimicrobial Therapy for Superficial Soft-Tissue infections
(continued)

Infection	Micro-organisms
Folliculitis, furuncles, carbuncles	*S aureus* (methicillin-susceptible *S aureus* [MSSA] or methicillin-resistant *S aureus* [MRSA])
Recurrent furunculosis	Check for nasal or perianal carrier of *S aureus.*
Whirlpool folliculitis	*P aeruginosa*

Therapy and Comments*

Warm saline compresses with or without topical anti-microbials are often sufficient for folliculitis.

Incision and drainage with or without topical antimicrobials often suffice for furuncles.

Oral: Antistaphylococcal penicillin, first-generation cephalosporin,*** clindamycin (300 mg q8h), levofloxacin (750 mg q.d.), moxifloxacin (400 mg q.d.)

For CA-MRSA, see impetigo.

IV: Antistaphylococcal penicillin, first-generation cephalosporin,*** clindamycin (600-900 mg q8h)

For MRSA: Vancomycin (15 mg/kg q12h), linezolid (600 mg q12h), daptomycin (4 mg/kg q24h); tigecycline (100 mg initial dose, then 50 mg q12h)

If nasal culture positive, nasal mupirocin (Bactroban®)

Oral: Antistaphylococcal penicillin, first-generation cephalosporin,*** clindamycin (300 mg q8h); or therapy for MRSA (see impetigo) possibly with rifampin (Rifadin®, Rimactane®) (300 mg b.i.d.)

Self-limiting; treatment is not necessary.

(continued on next page)

Table 4-1: Common Microbial Etiology and Antimicrobial Therapy for Superficial Soft-Tissue Infections *(continued)*

Infection	Micro-organisms
Hidradenitis suppurativa	Acute: *S aureus*
	Chronic: *S aureus*, *Enterobacteriaceae*, *Pseudomonas* spp., anaerobes

CA-MRSA=community-acquired MRSA; MRSA=methicillin-resistant *S aureus*; MSSA=methicillin-susceptible *S aureus*.

*Doses are based on normal renal and hepatic function.

Duration of therapy of most superficial skin infections is 7 to 10 days. One recent study of cellulites in immunocompetent hosts found 5 days was effective for uncomplicated infections.

**Oral antistaphylococcal penicillins include cloxacillin (Cloxapen®) (250-500 mg q6h) and dicloxacillin (Dynapen®) (250-500 mg q6h; parenteral antistaphylococcal penicillins include oxacillin (Bactocill®) (0.5-2 g q4-6h), nafcillin (Nafcil®) (0.5-2 g q4-6h)

Furuncle/Carbuncle

If folliculitis extends beyond the hair follicle into subcutaneous tissues, a furuncle may result. A furuncle is a deeper inflammatory nodule that often follows folliculitis. Furuncles usually measure <0.5 mm in diameter (Figure 4-3, see color plate insert). A carbuncle is a larger, deeper,

Therapy and Comments*

Antistaphylococcal agents for MSSA or MRSA based on susceptibility

Empirical: β-lactam/β-lactamase inhibitor,‡ cefoxitin (1-2 g q6H), cefotetan (0.5-1 g q12h), carbapenem***; clindamycin (600-900 mg t.i.d.) plus fluoroquinolone (ciprofloxacin, [Cipro®, ProQuin® XR] 750 mg q12h orally/400 mg q8-12h IV, or levofloxacin 750 mg q24h)

***Oral first-generation cephalosporins include cephalexin (Keflex®) (250-500 mg q6h) and cefadroxil (Duricef®, Ultracef®) (250-500 mg q12h); parenteral first-generation cephalosporins include cephalothin (0.5-2 g q4-6h) and cefazolin (Ancef®, Kefzol®) (0.5-1 g q8h).

†Erythromycin (250-500 mg q6h), azithromycin (Zithromax®) (500 mg on day 1, followed by 250 mg q.d.), clarithromycin (Biaxin®, Biaxin® XL) (500 mg q12 or 1 g XL q.d.)

‡Oral β-lactam/β-lactamase inhibitors include amoxicillin/clavulanate (Augmentin®, Augmentin® XR) (875/125 mg q12h), parenteral β-lactam/β-lactamase inhibitors include ampicillin/sulbactam (Unasyn®) (1.5-3 g q6h), ticarcillin/clavulanate (Timentin®) (3.1 g q4-6h), piperacillin/tazobactam (Zosyn® IV) (3.375 g-4.5 g q6h)

4

indurated, more serious lesion that often occurs as a confluent infection consisting of multiple furuncles (Figure 4-4, see color plate insert).

Furuncles and carbuncles often arise when areas of skin containing hair follicles are exposed to friction and perspiration. The back of the neck, face, axillae, and buttocks are commonly involved. Factors that predispose patients to the development of these lesions include obesity, corticosteroid therapy, and defective neutrophil function.

Outbreaks of furunculosis have been described often in high school athletes, particularly those with a history of skin injury. In addition, exposure to friends with furuncles appears to increase the risk of furunculosis independent of skin injury. Outbreaks involving multiple family members support the hypothesis that close contact with individuals with furunculosis is a risk factor for development of the disease.

S aureus is the most common cause of furunculosis and/or carbuncles. As described by Vugia and colleagues, outbreaks of *Mycobacterium furunculosis* affected customers using whirlpool footbaths at nail salons. *Mycobacterium fortuitum* and *Mycobacterium mageritense* were recovered from the footbaths and patient lesions.

Carbuncles often occur on the back of the neck, the back, or the thighs. Both furuncles and carbuncles begin as erythematous, firm, and tender nodular lesions that progress to a fluctuant mass that may drain pus spontaneously. *S aureus* most often is associated with furunculosis and carbunculosis. Furuncles occur in skin areas that contain hair follicles and that are subject to friction and perspiration (ie, neck, face, axillae, buttocks). Predisposing factors include obesity, corticosteroid use, defects in neutrophil function, and, probably, diabetes. Fever and malaise are frequent, and sepsis can occur. Blood-stream infection may occur with carbuncles (less so with furuncles), which may result in metastatic foci of infection (eg, endocarditis, osteomyelitis). *S aureus* in furuncles on the upper lip and nose may spread infection via emissary veins to the sinuses, resulting in cavernous sinus infection.

Impetigo

Impetigo is a vesiculopustular, superficial, intraepithelial infection of the skin that later becomes crusted. Impetigo generally occurs just beneath the stratum corium and is usually not associated with any systemic manifestations of infection. The disease starts as vesicular lesions that rapidly become pustular and crusty (Figure 4-5, see color plate insert).

Impetigo is most common in children and may be associated with poststreptococcal glomerulonephritis, although this condition is rare. Impetigo also occurs in adults, particularly if affected children share the same household.

The infection usually occurs in warm, humid conditions. Poverty, crowding, close contact (eg, between classmates, athletes, soldiers), and poor personal hygiene promote impetigo, which is easily spread within families and other closely associated groups of people. Infection typically arises at the site of minor skin trauma, such as insect bites or abrasions; distinguishing an insect bite from impetigo can be difficult. In addition, impetigo can be misdiagnosed as contact dermatitis. Carriage of GAS and *S aureus* predisposes one to subsequent impetigo.

S aureus and β-hemolytic *Streptococcus*, alone or in combination, are most commonly associated with impetigo. Impetigo manifests in two forms—bullous and nonbullous.

Mixtures of GAS and *S aureus* are isolated from about 50% of patients with nonbullous impetigo. Mixed flora of anaerobic *Streptococcus* with *Prevotella* or *Fusobacterium* species can sometimes be found in infections of the head and neck, while enteric gram-negative bacilli often mixed with *Bacteroides fragilis* can be isolated from infection of the buttocks. Nongroup A (ie, groups B, C, and G) *Streptococcus* has also been isolated from cases of nonbullous impetigo. A honey-colored crust over slightly erythematous areas of inflammation is characteristic. Regional lymphadenopathy without systemic symptoms is also common.

Bullous impetigo is primarily a staphylococcal infection. Bullous impetigo, most often seen in newborns and younger children, is due to *S aureus*, and accounts for <30%

of all impetigo cases. Bullous lesions develop rapidly and then drain, leaving thin, nonpurulent crusts overlying the involved skin areas. Lymphadenopathy is less prominent in bullous impetigo than in the more common vesiculo-pustular form.

Similar to the nonbullous form, the lesions appear vesicular initially but progress into flaccid, bullous lesions filled with yellow fluid. When these lesions rupture, light brown crusts form. The crusts and bullous lesions are characteristic of the infection. Regional lymphadenopathy is found less commonly in the bullous form. Fever and constitutional symptoms are uncommon in both disorders.

The early vesicular lesions may resemble the initial lesions of varicella or herpes simplex. However, the crusts of viral infections are usually harder. Impetigo occurs primarily in young children during the warm, humid months. Predisposing conditions include minor trauma, insect bites, poor hygiene, and pre-existing skin disease. The spread of impetigo is common within families by direct contact with infectious material. Culture may be obtained by removing the crust with sterile saline and culturing the surface of the lesion. Glomerulonephritis may follow impetigo caused by GAS, although this is now rare.

Cellulitis

Cellulitis is a diffuse and nonsuppurative infection of the skin and subcutaneous tissues. Predisposition to or risk factors for the development of cellulitis include disruption of the cutaneous barrier (eg, leg ulcer, traumatic wound, dermatoses, particularly tinea pedis), venous or lymphatic compromise (eg, venous insufficiency, stasis dermatitis, obesity, prior saphenectomy, previous tibial fracture, pregnancy), and previous history of cellulitis. In one prospective case-control study of adults conducted by Bjomsdottir and associates, the presence of S $aureus$ or β-hemolytic streptococci in the toe webs was significantly associated with acute cellulitis of the lower limbs.

S aureus and β-hemolytic *Streptococcus* are most commonly associated with cellulitis. A variety of other microorganisms produce cellulitis uncommonly and generally in specialized situations. As an example, *H influenzae* in children used to produce facial cellulitis or erysipelas until routine immunization against this organism began. Facial cellulitis still occurs, especially in children younger than 36 months; the pneumococcus is responsible for a number of these cases, particularly in children at risk for pneumococcal bacteremia. There is an increasing incidence of community-acquired methicillin-resistant *S aureus* (CA-MRSA), which primarily cause skin and soft-tissue infections (see Treatment below). *P aeruginosa* can cause cellulitis following a puncture wound, which may also produce complicating osteomyelitis. *Aeromonas hydrophilia*, *Vibrio vulnificus,* and a number of other pathogens can lead to cellulitis after exposure to fresh or seawater. Animal exposure, especially dog or cat bites, can lead to cellulitis due to specific organisms, such as *Pasteurella multocida* and *Erysipelothrix* (see Chapter 5).

The microbiology of cellulitis and its correlation to the site of infection were investigated in >200 swab and 64 needle-aspirate specimens, as shown in Brook. The highest recovery of anaerobic bacteria was from the neck, trunk, groin, external genitalia, and legs. Aerobes outnumbered anaerobes in the arms and hands. The predominant aerobes were *S aureus*, GAS, and *Escherichia coli*. *Peptostreptococcus*, *B fragilis* group, *Prevotella* species, and *Clostridium* species were the predominant anaerobes. Certain clinical findings correlated with the following pathogens: swelling and tenderness with *Clostridium* species, *S aureus*, and GAS; regional adenopathy with *B fragilis*; gangrene and necrosis with anaerobes with *Enterobacteriaceae*; and foul odor or gas in the tissues with anaerobes.

Cellulitis lesions are typically red, warm, swollen, and tender (Figures 4-6 and 4-7, see color plate insert). The borders of the lesions are usually not clearly demarcated.

Previous trauma (ie, laceration, abrasion) may precede the development of cellulitis. Within days of the trauma, local tenderness, pain, and erythema develop. Fevers, chills, malaise, and regional lymphadenitis commonly accompany the infection. If left untreated, local abscesses can develop; areas of overlying skin necrosis may also occur. Therefore, cellulitis may be mistaken for a number of other clinical disorders, including deep-vein thrombosis (DVT), erythema nodosum, allergic reactions, insect bite reactions, or reactions to chemical irritants.

In some patients, the onset of symptoms can be abrupt with fever >40°C and pronounced rigors, which may be prolonged (>15 minutes). Severe myalgias and fatigue can occasionally mimic influenza, particularly if there is a delay in onset or in the recognition of local findings. Disorientation or mental status changes can occur in the absence of shock, particularly in the elderly.

Recurrent Cellulitis

A frustrating problem for some patients is recurrent cellulitis at sites of previous surgery (Figure 4-8, see color plate insert). This has been particularly associated with saphenous venectomy for coronary bypass surgery, after varicose vein stripping, and after procedures that affect lymphatic drainage (as from radical mastectomy, neoplasia, or radiation therapy). Patients may experience acute pain, fever, and erythema at the site of the surgical scar. Tinea pedis is often an associated finding, although we reported an instance associated with underlying psoriasis. Although pathogens commonly have not been isolated in this form of cellulitis, some researchers suggest that an underlying skin disorder, such as tinea pedis, predisposes a patient to invasion with *Streptococcus* species. Cellulitis is often recurrent if the underlying skin disorder is not controlled. Similarly, recurrent cellulitis has occurred in patients after radical mastectomy. Among patients with recurrent episodes of lower extremity cellulitis and no obvious portal of entry, anal colonization with group G *Streptococcus* and possibly GAS and other β-hemolytic streptococci may constitute a reservoir for infection.

Erysipelas

Erysipelas is a distinctive form of cellulitis involving the superficial epidermis. Erysipelas differs from cellulitis in that the lesion is indurated, scarlet red with a well-demarcated border, usually painful, and often complicated by lymphangitis. Erysipelas is more common in children and older adults (Figures 4-9a and 4-9b, see color plate insert). The face and lower extremities are the sites of most frequent involvement. Because erysipelas produces lymphatic obstruction, it tends to recur in the same area. Occasionally, the infection extends more deeply, producing cellulitis. Subcutaneous abscess and necrosis are rarely described. Fever and systemic symptoms occur in most cases, while bacteremia is found in approximately 5% of patients. Patients who have venous insufficiency or lymphatic insufficiency (ie, recurrent cellulitis after venectomy or radical mastectomy) have had a high relapse rate. These lesions should be differentiated from erythema nodosum, shingles, erysipelothrix infection, and skin lesions of Lyme disease.

Hidradenitis Suppurativa

Hidradenitis suppurativa is a suppurative disease of the apocrine glands, usually in the axillary, genital, breast, or perianal areas. Affected patients may present with acute abscesses, but the condition often progresses to a chronic state with persistent pain, fistula formation, purulent drainage, and dermal scarring.

Although the precise pathophysiology of hidradenitis suppurativa is unclear, it is generally thought that occlusion of the apocrine or follicular ducts leading to ductal dilitation and stasis is the initiating event. Bacteria can enter the glands through the hair follicles and subsequently multiply in the environment of the obstructed sweat of the blocked apocrine gland. In the axilla, *S aureus* and streptococci are the most common pathogens in the initial stage of infection. Other organisms may be identified, such as gram-negative bacilli and anaerobes, when the disease advances to its later stages. In hidradenitis suppurativa in the perianal region, there is increased incidence of *Streptococcus milleri* and *Bacteroides* species.

Because the apocrine glands do not become active until puberty, it is rare to experience hidradenitis suppurativa before the onset of puberty. Patients with acne are especially susceptible. The disease affects both sexes, and the incidence is higher in blacks than in whites. There is no significant association with shaving habits, deodorant use, or the application of chemical depilatory agents.

Hidradenitis suppurativa initially presents with deep-seated nodules that tend to coalesce, resulting in acute abscesses and surrounding tissue inflammation. Eventually, the coalesced abscesses discharge through multiple openings, triggering progressive destruction of normal skin architecture with dermal and subcutaneous fibrosis. Chronic hidradenitis suppurativa is characterized by recurrent disease, often starting during adolescence (Figure 4-10, see color plate insert). The lesions are usually bilateral and vary from few to many. Ultimately, chronic sinus tract infections develop with intermittent drainage and cicatricial scarring. In some patients, infection is associated with cellulitis of the scalp (acne conglobata); in such cases, a distinctive spondyloarthropathy may occur.

Treatment of hidradenitis suppurativa is often difficult and extremely frustrating. Therapy consists primarily of antibiotics (usually broad spectrum for mixed infections) and simple measures, such as local warm compresses for early disease. Topical synthetic retinoids and intralesional administration of steroids have been tried with variable results for both subacute and chronic disease. Controversy exists regarding the most appropriate surgical approach in the management of hidradenitis suppurativa. Local incision and drainage of individual pustules or abscesses is often required in the acute phase, but incision and drainage may not prevent recurrent episodes of the disease. Many experts recommend that early isolated lesions be excised rather than drained because excision reduces the chance of extensive scarring. Deroofing of sinus tracts, which may be partially epithelialized, may be more definitive in preventing progressive disease when fistulous tracts have occurred. When the disease has become chronic and extensive, most experts recommend removal of the affected area and the adjacent apocrine glandular zone, with wide excision of the affected area, allowing the wound to heal by secondary intention. Skin grafting may be required. Concomitant treatment with antimicrobial agents that have both aerobic and anaerobic spectra is recommended. Several β-lactamase inhibitor combinations, such as amoxicillin/clavulanate (Augmentin®, Augmentin® XR), ampicillin/sulbactam (Unasyn®), ticarcillin/clavulanate (Timentin®), and piperacillin/tazobactam (Zosyn®IV), should provide an appropriate spectrum of coverage for this mixed infection. When the lesions are multiple and extensive, we recommend plastic surgery consultation for extensive excision with skin graft or flap to cover the area.

Diagnosis

Diagnosis of pyodermas is usually made clinically, based on its manifestations. Although the skin is easily accessible for culture, isolation of an infecting organism has not been consistent, usually because of the presence of contaminated normal skin flora. In addition, because certain skin lesions are caused by bacterial products or toxins rather than by bacteria themselves, the number of bacteria at the infection site may be too few to be cultured consistently. Therefore, the etiologic diagnosis and management of bacterial skin infections, especially in an office setting, are frequently based on clinical presentation and less commonly on microbiologic cultures. In patients who have skin and soft-tissue infections that require hospitalization, a more aggressive approach is needed to identify the etiologic agent because many of these patients have failed outpatient therapy. Outpatient therapy fails because of misdiagnosis, the wrong choice of therapy, or noncompliance. Culture of folliculitis, furunculosis, carbunculosis, impetigo, and hidradenitis suppurativa should usually yield the etiology. Although staphylococci are frequently found, certain special circumstances suggest consideration of other organisms. Exposure to hot tubs should alert physicians to the possible role of *P aeruginosa*, and patients who have *Candida* folliculitis may have a systemic *Candida* infection. Culture of impetigo may be obtained by removing the superficial crust with sterile saline and culturing the surface of the lesion. Blood culture is usually not helpful, but it would be appropriate in patients with systemic manifestations of disease and carbuncles because they may have bacteremia.

Numerous studies have evaluated the utility of intradermal needle aspirations in the bacteriologic diagnosis of cellulitis, but the issue remains controversial. Recent studies have reported rates of isolation of pathogenic organisms ranging from 5% to 36%. The most common pathogens isolated from needle-aspirate studies are staphylococci and streptococci. The method of needle aspiration is similar in most of these studies. First, the site of aspiration is cleansed with povidone-iodine solution and the skin over the area is punctured, without prior anesthesia, with a 22-gauge needle attached to a disposable plastic syringe. The contents of the syringe, previously filled with 1 mL of sterile isotonic saline, are injected subcutaneously. The fluid is then aspirated, with the needle still inserted in the subcutaneous tissue. Aspirated material is promptly taken to the microbiology laboratory and inoculated immediately into culture medium. Needle aspiration is not recommended for most cases of pyodermas, but it may be appropriate in selected cases when treatment fails or when the patient is immunosuppressed. In patients with cellulitis but without a localized primary infection such as a furuncle, streptococci can be identified by fluorescence microscopy in about 70% of patients, although cultures are frequently negative.

Treatment

When a patient presents with a skin or soft-tissue infection, an initial consideration of therapy is whether the infection is severe enough to warrant hospital admission. Most pyodermas do not trigger systemic symptoms and can be managed in the outpatient setting using oral antimicrobial agents. There are no well-documented criteria for the decision about site of care (ie, outpatient vs inpatient therapy). However, hospitalization should be considered based on these factors: severity of illness (ie, abnormality of vital signs and extent of soft-tissue involvement, see Chapter 7); patient's age; presence of comorbid conditions that can be affected by an acute infection (ie, diabetes, congestive heart failure [CHF]); and the need for close observation or surgical management.

According to Stevens and colleagues (2005), the recently published Infectious Diseases Society of America (IDSA) guidelines on the management of skin infections recommend that patients with soft-tissue infections accompanied by signs and symptoms of systemic toxicity (eg, fever or hypothermia, tachycardia [heart rate >100 beats/min], hypotension [systolic blood pressure <90 or 20 mm Hg below baseline] have blood drawn for the following laboratory tests: blood culture and susceptibilities, complete blood count (CBC) with differential, creatinine, bicarbonate, creatinine phosphokinase (CPK), and C-reactive protein (CRP). In those patients with hypotension and/or elevated creatinine levels, low serum bicarbonate, elevated CPK (ie, two to three times normal), marked left shift, or CRP >13 mg/L, hospitalization should be considered and a definitive etiologic diagnosis aggressively pursued, including procedures such as needle aspiration or punch biopsy for Gram stain and culture as well as requests for a surgical consultation for inspection, exploration, and/or drainage. Other clues to potentially severe deep soft-tissue infection include (1) pain disproportionate to the physical findings, (2) violaceous bullae, (3) cutaneous hemorrhage, (4) skin sloughing, (5) skin anesthesia, (6) rapid progression, and (7) gas in the tissue (see Chapter 8). In these cases, emergent surgical evaluation is of paramount importance for both diagnostic and therapeutic reasons.

When the decision to hospitalize is made, clinicians must determine the extent of infection, the presence of devitalized tissues, the state of vascular supply, the patient's immune and nutritional status, the etiologic agent, and the antimicrobial susceptibility pattern. In addition, the option of timely surgical intervention should be considered in cases of deep infections.

Antimicrobial therapy plays an important part in the treatment of skin and soft-tissue infections. Frequently, the etiologic agent is not known when therapy is initiated. Table 4-1 lists our recommendations for the treatment of bacterial pyodermas. For uncomplicated folliculitis, local measures, including warm compresses and topical antimicrobials such as mupirocin (Bactroban®, Centany™), are usually sufficient. For other infections, oral agents that have a spectrum of activity against common infecting organisms, such as *Staphylococcus* or *Streptococcus*, are preferred for outpatients. In uncomplicated cellulitis, 5 days of antibiotic treatment is as effective as 10 days.

Antibiotic treatment alone is effective in most patients with cellulitis. However, patients who are slow to respond may have a deeper infection or underlying conditions such as diabetes, chronic venous insufficiency, or lymphedema. In some patients, cutaneous inflammation sometimes worsens after initiating therapy, probably because the sudden destruction of pathogens releases potent enzymes that increase local inflammation. Elevation of the affected area, an important and often neglected aspect of treatment, quickens improvement by promoting gravity drainage of the edema and inflammatory substances. Patients should also receive appropriate therapy for any underlying condition that may have predisposed them to the infection (ie, tinea pedis, venous eczema [stasis dermatitis], trauma).

Treatment of recurrent furunculosis has been more frustrating. This infection is commonly found in patients who are chronic carriers of *S aureus* in the nares, anus, or both. The infection results from self-inoculation. The goal of therapy is to reduce or eradicate *S aureus* from the carrier. Antiseptic soaps or shampoo reduce the total population density of staphylococci. Local application of bacitracin (Neosporin®, Polysporin®) or mupirocin ointment to the anterior nares and anus may be helpful. An oral antistaphylococcal β-lactam agent alone (ie, dicloxacillin, cephalexin) is effective for acute attacks, but none has been shown to reduce recurrences. However, combining this type of agent with rifampin has been successful (Table 4-2).

In hospitalized patients, empiric antimicrobial therapy should be initiated to treat or prevent life-threatening infections. Therefore, the ideal agent or agents should cover the most common pathogens associated with life-threatening skin infections. β-lactam/β-lactamase inhibitor combinations, carbapenems, and combinations that have activity against staphylococci, streptococci, aerobic gram-negative rods, and anaerobic organisms have been shown to be consistently successful.

Of increasing concern is the emergence of antimicrobial resistance among isolates of CA-MRSA that are associated with skin infections (see Chapter 3). In the past, MRSA was usually limited to patients who were in the hospital (hospital-acquired methicillin-resistant *S aureus* [HA-MRSA]) or resided in a long-term care facility. Recently, outbreaks of skin infections caused by CA-MRSA have occurred among

Table 4-2: Approach to the Patient With Recurrent Staphylococcal Furunculosis

Acute

- Antistaphylococcal oral antibiotics (dicloxacillin or cloxacillin, 250-500 mg q6h; amoxicillin/clavulanate, 500-875 mg q12h; first-generation cephalosporin; clindamycin,150-300 mg q8h); levofloxacin 500 mg q.d., moxifloxacin 400 mg q.d.

- If large and fluctuant (eg, abscess or carbuncle), drain surgically

Recurrent

- Treat acute infection as above

- Meticulous skin care
  - Use antibacterial soaps (eg, pHisoderm®) and wash frequently.
  - Use topical antibiotics to treat superficial abrasions (bacitracin, mupirocin, neomycin).
  - Keep draining lesions covered to prevent secondary infections.

- Eradication of carrier state: if recurrent infection continues, try combination of:
  - Rifampin (300 mg q12h) *plus* TMP/SMX (160/800 mg q12h), dicloxacilllin (500 mg q6h), first-generation cephalosporin, minocycline (100 mg q12h), or clindamycin (150-300 mg q8h) for 10 to 14 d

---

prison and jail inmates, intravenous drug users, gay men, participants in contact sports, and children. However, there are now enough cases in patients without these risk factors so that CA-MRSA needs to be considered in all patients with skin infections. This has increased the importance of obtaining cultures of even mild skin infections. In general, CA-MRSA strains are usually susceptible in vitro to trimethoprim/sulfamethoxazole (TMP/SMX) (Bactrim™, Septra®) and minocycline (Minocin®) or doxycycline (Doryx®, Monodox®, Vibramycin®), and these agents can usually be used for mild-to-moderate infections. In addition, they are often susceptible to clindamycin, but, if considering the agent, isolates resistant to erythromycin and sensitive to clindamycin should be evaluated for inducible clindamycin resistance using the D test. Clinicians are advised to consult their reference laboratory to determine if D testing is routine or must be requested. If inducible resistance is present, an alternative agent is recommended. The newer fluoroquinolones, such as levofloxacin (Levaquin®) and moxifloxacin (Avelox®) usually have good activity for methicillin-susceptible S aureus (MSSA) but are generally not effective for MRSA. If active in vitro, oral rifampin (Rifadin®, Rimactane®) can be added for antimicrobial efficacy, but it should never be used as monotherapy because of the possibility of rapid emergence of resistance.

At present, the only US Food and Drug Administration (FDA)-approved antimicrobials for MRSA are parenterally administered vancomycin (Vancocin®) (although rare isolates of vancomycin-intermediate MRSA [VISA] strains have been recently described), quinupristin/dalfopristin (Synercid®), linezolid (Zyvox®), daptomycin (Cubicin®), and tigecycline (Tygacil®). Of these, only linezolid is available by oral administration. Agents effective for MRSA that are under development, or not yet marketed at the time of this writing, include the lipoglycopeptides televancin, dalbavancin, and oritavancin; the penicillin-binding protein 2a (PBP-2a)-targeted β-lactams ceftobiprole and ceftaroline, and a folic acid inhibitor iclaprim (see Chapter 3).

Persistent pustular skin infections that do not respond to oral β-lactam therapy are increasingly likely to be caused by MRSA. Such lesions should be cultured and antibiotic susceptibilities determined. Fluctuant lesions should be drained. An agent to which the isolate is susceptible should be used. For mild infections, oral agents, such as TMP/SMX, doxycycline, or clindamycin, can be considered. One caveat concerning TMP/SMX, however, is that it does not adequately cover for *S pyogenes;* therefore, if *S pyogenes* is also likely, an alternative agent or combination with penicillin is recommended. For serious infections requiring hospitalization, vancomycin, linezolid, or daptomycin are effective.

Surgical intervention is usually not required for pyodermas, but its role cannot be overestimated in cases of deeper infections or necrotizing skin infections (see Chapter 7). For furuncles, carbuncles, and hidradenitis suppurativa, however, surgical drainage is indicated if the lesions are large and fluctuant. Antibiotic treatment is indicated for abcesses >4.5 cm or if systemic signs of infection are present, and treatment should be continued until evidence of acute inflammation has subsided.

Treatment of hidradenitis suppurativa can be difficult, particularly when the infection is chronic, because of deep-seated abscesses and scar tissue that are inaccessible to antimicrobial agents. Antimicrobial therapy with local moist heat is often helpful in the initial phases of infection. Surgical drainage is required in the management of abscesses. Radical excision of tissue with subsequent skin grafting is often necessary for severe cases of extensive scarring.

Prevention

Management of patients with recurrent furunculosis presents a troublesome problem. Most patients do not have definable underlying defects. However, a higher rate of nasal colonization with *S aureus* has been observed in subgroups of patients (ie, diabetic patients, dialysis patients). Even small scratches or blisters can be colonized more rapidly and infected early in such patients. Therefore, we recommend the use of topical antibiotics (such as bacitracin, mupirocin, or neomycin) for early treatment of abrasions in these patients. In one study comparing the efficacy of topical mupirocin 2% cream with oral cephalexin in the therapy of secondarily infected traumatic skin lesions (eg, lacerations), pathogen eradication rates in the evaluated patients were 100% for both treatment groups.

Preventive management of recurrent furunculosis involves several measures (Table 4-2):

1. Meticulous skin care using antibacterial soaps (eg, hexachlorophene [pHisoHex®], chlorhexidine [Hibiclens®]) and washing frequently. Because infections (particularly impetigo) may be spread among family members, a separate towel and washcloth (carefully washed in hot water before use) should be reserved for each patient. Chlorhexidine or hexachlorophene solutions may also be used to reduce staphylococcal skin colonization.

2. Systemic antibiotic treatment should be administered for each active infection. Prolonged treatment (ie, 2 months) appears to be no more effective than a 10- to 14-day course in preventing recurrences.

3. Further measures aimed at elimination of a carrier state can be considered if recurrent infection continues. Nasal application of 2% mupirocin ointment in a white soft paraffin base for 5 days can eliminate *S aureus* colonization in healthy patients for up to 90 days. Oral antibiotics, such as rifampin (with another antimicrobial to prevent resistance), can be used to try to eradicate a carrier state. In one limited study, prophylaxis with oral clindamycin (Cleocin®, 150 mg once daily for 3 months) without an accompanying intranasal antimicrobial agent, reduced the frequency of recurrent staphylococcal skin infections.

Recurrent cellulitis in sites of previous surgery (ie, postcoronary artery bypass surgery or mastectomy) can also be prevented by reducing skin colonization using antibacterial soaps and by controlling tinea pedis in recurrent lower extremity cellulitis after coronary artery bypass surgery.

Prolonged antimicrobial prophylaxis with erythromycin has been shown to be effective and safe in these patients by preventing subsequent recurrent episodes of soft-tissue infections. We recommend, however, that systemic antibiotics be reserved only for patients who do not respond to antibacterial soaps and for control of tinea pedis in recurrent lower extremity cellulitis.

Selected Readings

Baddour LM, Bisno AL: Recurrent cellulitis after saphenous venectomy for coronary bypass. *Ann Intern Med* 1982;97:493-496.

Bisno AL, Stevens DL: Streptococcal infections of skin and soft tissues. *N Engl J Med* 1996;334:240-245.

Bjornsdottir S, Gottfredsson M, Thorisdottir AS, et al: Risk factors for acute cellulitis of the lower limb: a prospective case-control study. *Clin Infect Dis* 2005;41:1416-1422.

Brook I: Cellulitis and fasciitis. *Curr Treat Options Infect Dis* 2000;2:127-146.

Brook I, Frazier EH: Aerobic and anaerobic microbiology of axillary hidradenitis suppurativa. *J Med Microbiol* 1999;48:103-105.

Brook I, Frazier EH: Clinical features and aerobic and anaerobic characteristics of cellulitis. *Arch Surg* 1995;130:786-792.

File TM Jr, Tan JS: Treatment of bacterial skin and soft tissue infections. *Surg Gynecol Obstet* 1991;172 (Suppl):17-24.

Finch R: Skin and soft tissues infections. *Lancet* 1988;1:164-168.

Henkel TJ, Bottonfield G, Drehobl M, et al: Comparison of mupirocin calcium cream with oral cephalexin in the treatment of secondarily infected traumatic lesions. 20th International Congress of Chemotherapy. Sydney, Australia, Abstract No. 5308, 1997.

Herold BC, Immergluck LC, Maranan MC, et al: Community-acquired methicillin-resistant *Staphylococcus aureus* in children with no identified predisposing risk. *JAMA* 1998;279;593-598.

Kars M, van Dijk H, Salimans MM, et al: Association of furunculosis and familial deficiency of mannose-binding lectin. *Eur J Clin Invest* 2005;35:531-534.

Klempner MS, Styrt B: Prevention of recurrent staphylococcal skin infections with low dose oral clindamycin therapy. *JAMA* 1988; 260:2682-2685.

Kremer M, Zuckerman R, Avraham Z, et al: Long-term antimicrobial therapy in the prevention of recurrent soft-tissue infections. *J Infect* 1991;22:37-40.

Lebre C, Girard-Pipau F, Roujeau JC, et al: Value of fine-needle aspiration in infectious cellulitis. *Arch Dermatol* 1996;132:842-843.

Moreno F, Crisp C, Jorgenson JH, et al: Methicillin-resistant *Staphylococcus aureus* as a community organism. *Clin Infect* 1995;21:1308-1312.

Newell PM, Norden CW: Value of needle aspiration in bacteriologic diagnosis of cellulitis in adults. *J Clin Microbiol* 1988;26: 401-404.

Parks RW, Parks TG: Pathogenesis, clinical features and management of hidradenitis suppurativa. *Ann R Coll Surg Engl* 1997;79:83-89.

Stevens DL, Bisno AL, Chambers HF, et al: Practice guidelines for the diagnosis and management of skin and soft-tissue infections. *Clin Infect Dis* 2005;41:1373-1406.

Stevens DL: Cellulitis, pyoderma, abscesses and other skin and subcutaneous infections. In: Cohen J, Powderly WG, et al, eds: *Infectious Diseases*, 2nd ed. Edinburgh, Scotland, Mosby, 2004, pp 133-144.

Swartz MN, Pasternack MS: Cellulitis and subcutaneous tissue infections. In: Mandell GL, Bennett JE, Dolin R, eds: *Principles and Practice of Infectious Diseases*, 6th ed. New York, NY, Churchill Livingstone, 2005, pp 1172-1193.

Vugia DJ, Jang Y, Zizek C, et al: Mycobacteria in nail salon whirlpool footbaths, California. *Emerg Infect Dis* 2005;11:616-618.

Swartz MN: Cellulitis and subcutaneous tissue infections. In: Mandell GL, Bennett JE, Dolin R, eds: *Principles and Practice of Infectious Diseases*, 5th ed. New York, NY, Churchill Livingstone, 2000, pp 1037-1057.

Waldvogel FA: *Staphylococcus aureus*. In: Mandell GL, Douglas RG Jr, Bennett JE, eds: *Principles and Practice of Infectious Diseases*, 4th ed. New York, NY, Churchill Livingstone, 1995, pp 1754-1776.

4

Chapter **5**

Skin Infections Associated With Underlying Conditions

Secondary Infections

Secondary infections develop in areas where skin is abnormal or already damaged. Although the bacteria of secondary infections do not necessarily produce the underlying skin disorder, their proliferation and subsequent invasion of surrounding areas can cause significant infection. Lesions that are associated with secondary infections include postoperative wounds, infections from trauma and bites, pressure ulcers, infected cysts, and diabetic foot ulcer infections (Table 5-1). This chapter examines these lesions, except for diabetic foot infections, which are reviewed separately in Chapter 6.

Surgical Site Infections

Surgical site infections (SSIs), also called postoperative wound infections, remain a major source of morbidity and mortality in surgical patients. Based on the type of surgical procedure and the patient's underlying condition, the overall incidence of postoperative wound infection ranges from 2% to 10%. SSIs account for 14% to 16% of all hospital-acquired infections. The incidence of hospital-acquired infections generally increases with the class of operative procedure, based on degree of contamination: clean operations, 2% to 5%; clean-contaminated, 10%; contaminated, 15%; and dirty, 25% to >30%.

SSIs are divided into the categories of superficial incisional SSIs, deep incisional SSIs, and organ/space SSIs.

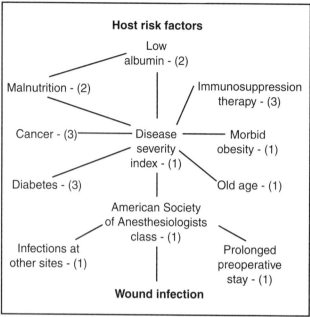

Figure 5-1: Relationship between host risk factors and surgical wound infection. Number in parentheses refers to likelihood of relationship. 1=definite; 2=likely; 3=possible. From Sherertz et al, *Am J Infect Control* 1992;20: 263-270.

Superficial incisional SSIs involve only the subcutaneous space between the skin and underlying muscular fascia; occur within 30 days of the index operation; and are documented with at least one of the following: (1) purulent incisional drainage; (2) positive culture of aseptically obtained fluid or tissue from the superficial wound; (3) local signs and symptoms of pain or tenderness, swelling, and erythema, and the incision is opened by the surgeon (unless culture-negative); or (4) diagnosis of SSI by the attending surgeon or physician.

Table 5-1: Skin Infections Associated With Underlying Conditions

Infection	Usual Pathogens
Surgical site	*Staphylococcus aureus*
	- MSSA
	- MRSA
	Mixed infection: *S aureus*, *Enterococcus*, Enterobacteriaceae, *Pseudomonas*, anaerobes
Recurrent cellulitis associated post venectomy for coronary artery bypass graft	β-hemolytic streptococcus (group C, F, G most common, occasionally Group A; *S aureus* may occur if associated with tinea pedis)
Bite wound	
• Dog, cat	*Pasteurella multocida*, *S aureus*, *Capnocytophaga canimorsus* (dog)

CA-MRSA=community-acquired methicillin-resistant *S aureus*; MRSA=methicillin-resistant *S aureus*; MSSA=methicillin-susceptible *S aureus*

Empiric Antimicrobial Therapy IV*

MSSA: Nafcillin (Nafcil®), cefazolin (Ancef®), clindamycin (Cleocin®), vancomycin, levofloxacin (Levaquin®), moxifloxacin (Avelox®); if concern for or documented MRSA: vancomycin, linezolid (Zyvox®), quinupristin/dalfopristin (Synercid®), daptomycin[4] (Cubicin®)

Cefoxitin,[1] cefotetan,[1] β-lactam/β-lactamase inhibitors: ampicillin/sulbactam (Unasyn®),[1] piperacillin/tazobactam (Zosyn®IV), ticarcillin/clavulanate (Timentin®), tigecycline (Tygacil®),[1,5] imipenem/cilastatin (Primaxin®), meropenem (Merrem®IV), ertapenem (Invanz®).[2] If allergic to β-lactam: tigecycline,[1,5] clindamycin, or metronidazole (Flagyl®) *plus* a fluoroquinolone (ie, ciprofloxacin [Cipro®, ProQuin® XR], levofloxacin[2]) 750 mg q.d. Use vancomycin or linezolid or daptomycin[4] if a concern for MRSA (dalbavancin and telavancin, pending approval by the FDA).

Penicillin, cephalosporin, macrolide, clindamycin (evaluate for tinea pedis and treat, if present; effective treatment may reduce recurrences.)

Amoxicillin/clavulanate (oral), ampicillin/sulbactam (IV); ceftoxitin, ertapenem; tigecycline,[1,5] doxycycline; clindamycin plus trimethoprim/sulfamethoxazole (TMP/SMX) (Bactrim™, Septra®) or a fluoroquinolone (levofloxacin, ciprofloxacin, moxifloxacin); consider CA-MRSA

(continued on next page)

Table 5-1: Skin Infections Associated With Underlying Conditions
(continued)

Infection	Usual Pathogens
Bite wound *(cont.)*	
• Human	*S aureus*, *Streptococcus* sp, anaerobes, *Eikenella corrodens*
Trauma infection	
• General	*Staphylococcus aureus*, *Streptococcus pyogenes*
• Associated with specific risk factors	
Fresh water injury	*Aeromonas hydrophila* *Plesiomonas shigelloides*
Salt water injury	*Vibrio vulnificus*
Soil	*Pseudomonas aeruginosa*, *Clostridium* sp
Butchers, abattoir workers	*Erysipelothrix rhusiopathiae*
Nail puncture of the foot	*Pseudomonas aeruginosa*

*PO when appropriate

Empiric Antimicrobial Therapy IV*

Amoxicillin/clavulanate (oral), ampicillin/sulbactam (IV); ceftoxitin, ertapenem; tigecycline,[1,5] doxycycline (Doryx®, Monodox®, Vibramycin®); clindamycin *plus* TMP/SMX or a fluoroquinolone (levofloxacin, ciprofloxacin, moxifloxacin); consider CA-MRSA

MSSA: nafcillin, cefazolin, clindamycin, levofloxacin, moxifloxacin

MRSA: vancomycin, linezolid, daptomycin[4] (dalbavancin and telavancin, pending approval by the FDA)

Fluoroquinolone (ie, ciprofloxacin, levofloxacin), piperacillin/tazobactam, ticarcillin/clavulanate, third- or fourth-generation cephalosporin, imipenem, meropenem

Fluoroquinolone (ie, ciprofloxacin, levofloxacin), ceftazidime, cefepime, TMP/SMX, doxycycline

Piperacillin/tazobactam, ticarcillin/clavulanate, imipenem, meropenem, ciprofloxacin, or levofloxacin 750 mg q.d. *plus* clindamycin, aminoglycoside *plus* clindamycin

Penicillin, ampicillin, third- or fourth-generation cephalosporin, fluoroquinolone (ie, ciprofloxacin, levofloxacin)

Piperacillin/tazobactam, ticarcillin/clavulanate; imipenem, meropenem, ciprofloxacin, or levofloxacin +/- clindamycin; aminoglycoside +/- clindamycin

(continued on next page)

Table 5-1: Skin Infections Associated With Underlying Conditions
(continued)

Infection	Usual Pathogens
Pressure (decubitus) ulcer	Superficial: *S aureus*, β-hemolytic *Streptococcus*
	Deep: same as above, plus *Enterococcus* sp, Enterobacteriaceae, *Pseudomonas aeruginosa*, anaerobes

[1]Ampicillin/sulbactam (Unasyn®), cefazolin (Ancef®), cefepime (Maxipime®), cefotaxime (Claforan®), cefotetan (Cefotan®), cefoxitin (Mefoxin®), ceftazidime (Tazicef®), ceftriaxone (Rocephin®), clindamycin (Cleocin®), daptomycin (Cubicin®), doxycycline (Doryx®, Monodox®, Vibramycin®), fluoroquinolones (Cipro®, Levaquin®, ProQuin® XR), imipenem/cilastatin (Primaxin®), linezolid (Zyvox®), meropenem (Merrem®IV), metronidazole (Flagyl®), nafcillin, piperacillin/tazobactam (Zosyn®IV), quinupristin/dalfopristin (Synercid®), ticarcillin/clavulanate (Timentin®), tigecycline (Tygacil®), vancomycin (Vancocin®)

[1]Not effective for *Pseudomonas*

[2]Levofloxacin (IV or PO) is approved at 500 mg q.d. for uncomplicated skin infections due to *S pyogenes* or *S aureus*, as well as at 750 mg q.d. (PO or IV) for complicated skin and skin-structure infections due to MSSA, *S pyogenes*, *E faecalis*, or *P mirabilis*.

[3]Moxifloxacin (Avelox®) 400 mg q.d. is approved for uncomplicated skin infections due to *S aureus* and *S pyogenes* and for complicated skin and skin-structure infections (cSSSIs) due to MSSA, *Escherichia coli*, *Klebsiella pneumoniae*, or *Enterobacter cloacae*.

Empiric Antimicrobial Therapy IV*

Same as for wound infection, *S aureus*—
see previous page

Same as for mixed surgical site infections (SSIs)—
see previous page

[4]Daptomycin (Cubicin®) is approved for the treatment of complicated skin and skin-structure infections caused by susceptible strains of the following gram-positive micro-organisms: *Staphylococcus aureus* (including methicillin-resistant strains), *Streptococcus pyogenes, Streptococcus agalactiae, Streptococcus dysgalactiae subsp. equisimilis,* and *Enterococcus faecalis* (vancomycin-susceptible strains).

[5]Tigecycline is approved for cSSSIs caused by *Escherichia coli, Enterococcus faecalis* (vancomycin-susceptible isolates), *S aureus* (methicillin-susceptible and -resistant isolates), *Streptococcus agalactiae, Streptococcus anginosus* group (includes *S anginosus, S intermedius,* and *S constellatus*), *Streptococcus pyogenes,* and *Bacteroides fragilis.*

*PO when appropriate

5

A deep incisional infection involves the deep layers of soft tissue in the incision (eg, fascia and muscle) and occurs within 30 days of the operation or within 1 year if a prosthesis was inserted and has the same findings as described for a superficial incisional SSI.

An organ/space SSI has the same time constraints and evidence for infection as a deep incisional SSI and involves any part of the anatomy (organs or spaces) other than the incision opened during the operation. Superficial and deep incisional SSIs are skin and soft-tissue infections that are discussed in this chapter.

Most wounds become infected in the operating room while the incisions are open. Numerous risk factors for postoperative SSIs have been identified and verified by clinical studies. Predisposition to SSIs appears to be related to impairment of host factors that regulate immune response and wound healing (Figure 5-1). These factors include age, nutritional status, diabetes, obesity, immuno-compromising diseases, presence of other infections, and duration of preoperative stay. The severity of underlying conditions is also a significant predictor of risk of SSI. In addition to host factors, numerous surgery-related factors are associated with postoperative wound infections, including duration of surgery, hair removal procedures, surgical techniques of individual surgeons, presence or absence of drains or packs, primary or secondary closure techniques, and the use of irrigation.

In a typical SSI case, manifestations of infection occur 5 or more days after surgery, but may occur up to 2 weeks after the procedure. Usually, there is edema and redness of the wound (Figure 5-2, see color plate insert), but the most common early sign is increased pain. Purulent drainage often occurs. Necrosis and spreading infection are uncommon, but are associated with more severe infection (Figure 5-3, see color plate insert). Rarely does any bacterial pathogen cause fever or clinical evidence of soft-tissue infection within the first 48 hours after an operation or injury. Infections that do occur in this timeframe are almost always due to *S pyogenes* or *Clostridium* species. Accordingly, fever or systemic signs during the first several postoperative days should be followed by direct examination of the wound to rule out signs suggestive of streptococcal or clostridial infection (eg, compatible organisms present on Gram stain). White blood cells may not be evident in most clostridial infection and in some early streptococcal infections. Another rare cause of early fever and systemic signs following operation is staphylococcal toxic shock syndrome (TSS). In these cases, the wound is often deceptively benign in appearance. Erythroderma occurs early, but not immediately, and desquamation occurs late. Fever, hypotension, abnormal hepatic and renal blood studies, and diarrhea may be early findings. Treatment is to open the incision, culture, and begin antistaphylococcal treatment.

The physical appearance of the incision probably provides the most reliable information to diagnose a SSI. Local signs of pain, swelling, erythema, and purulent drainage are usually present. In morbidly obese patients or in those with deep, multilayer wounds such as after a thoracotomy, the external signs of SSI may become apparent very late but essentially always appear. While many patients with a SSI will have fever, it usually does not occur immediately postoperatively, and in fact, most postoperative fevers are not associated with a SSI. Flat, erythematous changes can occur around or near a surgical incision during the first week without swelling or wound drainage. Most resolve without any treatment, including antibiotics. The cause is unknown, but may relate to tape sensitivity or other local tissue insult not involving bacteria.

The most common pathogens associated with SSIs are *Staphylococcus* species, *Streptococcus* species, Enterobacteriaceae, *Pseudomonas aeruginosa*, and a number of other gram-negative organisms. Specific pathogens vary from one hospital to another. When postoperative wound infection is suspected, every attempt should be made

Table 5-2: Antibiotic Choices for Incisional Surgical Site Infections

Intestinal or Genital Tract Operations

Single Agents:	Combination Agents:
• Cefoxitin	• Facultative and aerobic activity
• Ceftizoxime (Cefizox®)	• Anaerobic activity
• Ampicillin/sulbactam	• Fluoroquinolone
• Ticarcillin/clavulanate	• Clindamycin
• Piperacillin/tazobactam	• Third-generation cephalosporin
• Imipenem/cilastatin	• Metronidazole*
• Meropenem	• Aztreonam (Azactam®)*
• Ertapenem	• Chloramphenicol
	• Aminoglycoside
	• Penicillin class + β-lactamase inhibitor

to provide an adequate path for drainage and to culture purulent drainage. Blood cultures are also indicated. Empiric antibiotic therapy should include coverage for the aforementioned pathogens based on the antimicrobial susceptibility patterns within the clinician's institution (Table 5-1). Once culture results are available, specific, pathogen-directed therapy should be used based on antimicrobial susceptibility.

Nonintestinal Operations

Trunk and Extremities Away from Axilla or Perineum:

- Oxacillin
- First-generation cephalosporin

Axillary or Perineum:

- Cefoxitin
- Ampicillin/sulbactam
- Others, as in Intestinal or Genital Tract Operations above

*Do not combine aztreonam with metronidazole because this combination has no activity against gram-positive cocci.

Adapted from Stevens et al, *Clin Infect Dis* 2005;41:1373-1406.

A common practice, endorsed by the Infectious Diseases Society of America (IDSA) guidelines for the diagnosis and management of skin and soft-tissue infections, is to open all infected wounds. If there is minimal surrounding evidence of invasive infection (>5 cm of erythema and induration), and if the patient has minimal systemic signs of infection (temperature <38.5° C, and pulse <100), antibiotics are unnecessary. Because incision and drainage of superficial abscesses rarely causes bacteremia, antibiotics are often not needed. For patients with temperatures >38.5° C or pulses >100, a short course of antibiotics, usually from 24 to 48 hours, may be indicated. The antibiotic choice is usually empiric, but can be supported by Gram stain and culture of the wound contents. A SSI following an operation on the intestinal tract or female genitalia has a high probability of a mixed gram-positive and -negative flora with both facultative and anaerobic organisms. If such an infection is being treated with empiric antibiotics, any antibiotic considered appropriate for treatment of intra-abdominal infection is reasonable (Table 5-2). If the operation was a clean procedure that did not enter the intestinal or genital tracts, *S aureus* (including MRSA) and streptococcal species are the most common organisms. Because incisions in the axilla have a significant recovery of gram-negative organisms, and those in the perineum have a higher incidence of gram-negative organisms and anaerobes, antibiotic choices should be made accordingly.

According to Bratzler, there is a strong national commitment to reduce SSIs through the implementation of the Surgical Infection Prevention and Surgical Care Improvement Projects. This initiative provides incentives and infrastructure for national data collection and quality improvement activities for hospitals on performance measures, such as appropriate use of prophylactic antimicrobials, blood-glucose monitoring for cardiac surgery, proper hair removal, and maintenance of normothermia in colorectal surgery.

Recurrent Cellulitis After Surgery

A frustrating problem for some patients is recurrent cellulitis in sites of previous surgery. This has been particularly associated after saphenous venectomy for coronary bypass surgery (see Figure 4-8, color plate insert), after varicose vein stripping, and after procedures that affect lymphatic drainage (such as from neoplasia, radiation therapy, or surgery). Patients may experience acute pain, fever, and erythema at the site of the surgical scar. Tinea pedis is often an associated finding, although other chronic skin disorders (ie, dermatitis, psoriasis) may also predispose to cellulitis. Although pathogens have not often been isolated in cellulitis, researchers have suggested that the underlying skin disorder, such as tinea pedis, predisposes to invasion with streptococcal species. Cellulitis often recurs if the underlying skin disorder is not controlled. Similarly, recurrent cellulitis has occurred in patients after radical mastectomy. See Chapter 4 for further discussion of therapy and prevention.

Bite Wound Infections

Dog and Cat Bite Wounds

Each year, more than 5 million Americans are bitten by animals. Approximately one half of all Americans will be bitten by an animal or by another person some time during their lives. An estimated 3% to 18% of dog bites and 28% to 80% of cat bites become infected. Dogs are responsible for most animal bite wounds, followed by cats, then by an unknown number of bites from exotic pets, small mammals, and nondomesticated animals. Infection after a dog bite usually manifests as cellulitis and is often associated with a discharge described as gray and malodorous. Wounds consist of tears, evulsions, punctures, and scratches. Septic arthritis is possible when the feline tooth penetrates a joint, especially of the hand (Figure 5-4, see color plate insert). Osteomyelitis and abscess formation can also result from such bites. Cats' teeth are slender and sharper than dogs' teeth, and they can easily penetrate into bones and joints, with proportionally increased rates of septic arthritis and osteomyelitis.

A wide range of aerobic and anaerobic organisms can cause bite wound infections. Inoculation of oral flora of the aggressor, or skin microbes from the victim, may occur during infliction of the bite, resulting in polymicrobial contamination and subsequent infection. In a study of infected

Table 5-3: Bacteria Isolated From Dog and Cat Bites

Bacteria	Dog Bite N=50	Cat Bite N=75
Aerobes		
Pasteurella sp	25 (50%)	43 (75%)
Streptococcus sp	23 (46%)	26 (46%)
S aureus	10 (20%)	2 (4%)
Coagulase-negative *Staphylococcus*	20 (42%)	25 (45%)
Neisseria sp	8 (16%)	11 (19%)
Corynebacterium sp	6 (12%)	16 (28%)
Moraxella sp	5 (10%)	20 (35%)
Enterococcus	5 (10%)	20 (35%)
Pseudomonas sp	3 (6%)	3 (5%)
Actinomyces sp	3 (6%)	2 (4%)
Enterobactcriaceae	9 (18%)	3 (5%)
Eikenella corrodens	1 (2%)	1 2%)
Anaerobes		
Fusobacterium sp	16 (32%)	19 (33%)
Bacteroides sp	15 (30%)	16 (28%)
Porphyromonas sp	14 (28%)	17 (30%)
Prevotella sp	14 (28%)	11 (19%)
Propionibacterium sp	10 (20%)	10 (18%)
Peptostreptococcus sp	8 (16%)	3 (5%)

From Talan DA, et al, *N Engl J Med* 1999;340:85-92.

cat and dog bite wounds, *Pasteurella* species, including *P multocida* and *P septica*, were the most common isolates, found in 75% of infected cat bites and in 50% of infected dog bites (Table 5-3). *Streptococcus*, *Staphylococcus*, *Moraxella*, *Corynebacterium*, and *Neisseria* were also commonly found. *S aureus* and *Streptococcus pyogenes*, which are part of the transient normal flora of human skin, and are uncommonly found in the oropharyngeal flora, were found relatively infrequently, especially in cat bites. This may result from the wounds being more heavily contaminated with oral zoonotic bacteria than with human skin flora. *Eikenella corrodens*, which is associated with human bite infections, was found in only one dog bite and one cat bite. Rarely, Enterobacteriaceae or *Pseudomonas* species are isolated. Anaerobes were also commonly isolated from infected dog or cat bite wounds, but they rarely occur. *Capnocytophaga canimorsus* has been associated with severe infection (often with disseminated intravascular coagulation and renal failure) in hosts compromised by previous splenectomy, severe liver disease, or other significant underlying immunosuppressant conditions. The fatality rate among these patients is approximately 25%.

5

Principles of management include careful medical examination of all puncture wounds, tears, and evulsions, as well as their proximity to blood vessels, nerves, tendons, bones, and joints. Patients who seek medical care after 8 to 12 hours of injury typically have established infection. The wounds may be nonpurulent (30% of dog bites; 42% of cat bites), purulent (58% of dog bites; 39% of cat bites), or abscesses (12% of dog bites; 19% of cat bites). If the wound is to the hand, careful examination of range of motion, nerve, and tendon function should be recorded. Appropriate management includes debridement, copious irrigation, selection of proper antimicrobial therapy, and elevation of the affected extremity, especially if there is edema. Cultures should only be obtained from infected or purulent wounds.

The findings of mixed aerobic/anaerobic pathogens in the wounds of infected bites suggest that empirical antimicrobial therapy should be directed against streptococci, staphylococci, anaerobes, and *Pasteurella* (for animal bites). *Pasteurella* species are usually susceptible to the penicillins, second- or third-generation cephalosporins, doxycycline, trimethoprim/sulfamethoxazole (TMP/SMX) (Bactrim™, Septra®), and the fluoroquinolones. Agents that may be typically used for routine skin infections—such as first-generation cephalosporins, clindamycin (Cleocin®), and erythromycin—are less active against *Pasteurella* in vitro and have been associated with clinical failures in cases where *Pasteurella* was cultured.

Empiric treatment of dog and cat bites is similar. Parenteral ampicillin/sulbactam (Unasyn®) or oral amoxicillin/clavulanate (Augmentin®, Augmentin®XR) will cover most of the spectrum of bite wound pathogens, including both aerobes (including *C canimorsus*) and anaerobes. Alternative antimicrobials that cover *P multocida*, methicillin-susceptible *S aureus* (MSSA), and the usual aerobic and anaerobic animal/human flora species include cefoxitin (Mefoxin®), piperacillin/tazobactam (Zosyn®IV), and carbenicillins such as ertapenem (Invanz®), imipenem/cilastatin (Primaxin®) and meropenem (Merrem®, Merrem®IV) intravenously and doxycycline (Doryx®, Monodox®, Vibramycin®) orally. Other regimens that could be used include fluoroquinolones (ciprofloxacin [Cipro®, ProQuin® XR], levofloxacin [Levaquin®], or moxifloxacin [Avelox®]) usually combined with metronidazole or clindamycin (Cleocin®). First-generation cephalosporins such as cephalexin (Keflex®), penicillinase-resistant penicillins (eg, dicloxacillin [Dynapen®]), macrolides (eg, erythromycin), and clindamycin, all have poor in vitro activity against *P multocida* and should be avoided as monotherapy. As for all skin infections, the possibility of CA-MRSA, which will affect antimicrobial therapy (see Chapter 3), must be considered.

Penicillin-allergic pregnant women comprise a special population because tetracyclines, sulfa compounds (in late pregnancy), and metronidazole are contraindicated. Similarly, the selection of an antimicrobial for penicillin-allergic children is problematic where tetracyclines and fluoroquinolones are contraindicated. In these situations, macrolides (eg, azithromycin 250 to 500 mg q.d. or clarithromycin 500 mg b.i.d. or extended release 1 g q.d.) are occasionally used; however, these patients should be followed closely and the potential increased risk of failure noted.

The duration of therapy varies by the severity of the injury or infection. Cellulitis and abscess often respond to 5 to 10 days of therapy. The therapy of early-presenting, noninfected wounds remains controversial. Wounds that are moderate to severe; have associated crush injury; have associated edema, either pre-existing or subsequent; wounds to the hands or in proximity to a bone or a joint; or wounds in compromised hosts should receive 3 to 5 days of prophylactic antimicrobial therapy. These wounds are often (85%) colonized with potential pathogens, and it is difficult to determine which will become infected.

All bite wounds should be irrigated with copious amounts (≥200 mL) of normal saline. If possible, puncture wounds should be irrigated with a high-pressure jet using a 20-mL syringe and an 18-gauge needle or catheter tip to access the wound. However, some puncture wounds are tiny and relatively inaccessible to irrigation. Appropriate wound irrigation may produce a 6- to 10-fold reduction in bite wound infection rates compared with bite wounds not receiving irrigation.

The most common error made in the treatment of bite wounds is failure to adequately debride and irrigate the wounds. Devitalized or necrotic tissue should be cautiously debrided, and foreign bodies and all other debris should be removed fastidiously from the wound. Appropriate and adequate anesthesia should be provided to make the procedure tolerable for the patient. Appropriate debridement decreased bite wound infection rates from 62% to 2% in one study.

Primary wound closure may be indicated for some uninfected wounds, especially facial wounds. However, closure of other types of bite wounds is not usually indicated. Wound edges should be approximated with adhesive strips in certain cases, and healing by secondary intention or by delayed closure may be indicated when infectious complications have been addressed.

A thorough history of the bite victim's immunization status should be obtained when the patient seeks treatment. Standard tetanus immunization guidelines should be followed in all circumstances, and appropriate vaccine or tetanus-immune globulin should be administered as required.

Infectious complications of bite wounds include septic arthritis, osteomyelitis, subcutaneous abscess formation, tendonitis, and rarely, bacteremia. Pain disproportionate to the severity of injury but located near a bone or joint should suggest periosteal penetration. Hand wounds are often more serious than those to fleshy parts of the body. These wound complications will necessitate prolonged therapy, such as 4 to 6 weeks for osteomyelitis and 3 to 4 weeks for synovitis. Noninfectious complications include nerve or tendon injury or severance, compartment syndrome, postinfectious and traumatic arthritis, fracture, and bleeding.

Human Bite Wounds

Human bites are usually more serious and more prone to infection and complication than those of animals (Figure 5-5, see color plate insert). Human bite wounds generally can be classified into three types: self-inflicted paronychia, occlusional bite wounds, and clenched-fist injuries. Self-inflicted paronychia may be the result of nail biting, thumb sucking, or similar activities. Occlusional bite wounds usually are intentionally inflicted injuries that occur during a physical confrontation. Clenched-fist injuries are unintentionally induced injuries occurring to the hand of an offensive-minded pugilist. Human bite wounds are the third most common type of bite wound encountered in emergency departments. Human bite wounds also may be sustained during sexual activity. Common locations for human bite wounds in children are the scalp and face, whereas the distal portion of the index or middle finger is the most common site for occlusional bite wounds. The ear, nose, forearm, breast, penis, scrotum, and vulva may be affected in adult bite wounds resulting from passionate or pugilistic activity. Clenched-fist injury usually produces a wound over the third, fourth, or fifth metacarpal head of the dominant hand. Any injury at this site is usually caused by an inadvertent human bite wound until proven otherwise. Patients with clenched-fist injuries often provide the physician with false information regarding the exact circumstances of the injury because of embarrassment or fear of legal ramifications. Bite wounds in children may be due to sports (look for imbedded teeth), but should also alert the clinician to possible child abuse. Approximately 60% to 70% of all human bite wounds are sustained to the hand and upper extremities, 15% to 20% to the head or neck, 10% to 20% to the trunk, and 5% to the lower extremities, with other sites accounting for the remaining 5% to 10% of human bite wounds.

Clenched-fist injuries are the most serious of human bite wounds and usually occur as a result of a fist striking the teeth of another. They are usually small, 3 to 5 mm, and generally are sustained on the knuckle of the dominant hand. Most of these wounds become infected, with swelling and discharge developing within hours of the injury.

Under healthy circumstances, the human mouth may harbor more than 40 species of bacteria. Almost 200 species of potentially pathogenic bacterial species have been described in the presence of gingivitis and periodontal disease. More than 50% of human bite wound infections contain mixed gram-negative and -positive bacteria. Anaerobes are found in more than 60% of human bite wounds, and it has been estimated that if sophisticated anaerobic culture techniques are used, up to 100% of human bite wounds may include anaerobic species.

The most common pathogens of human bites include *S aureus*, *Haemophilus influenzae*, and β-lactamase-producing oral anaerobic bacteria. In addition, *E corrodens* is found in 25% of clenched-fist injuries.

Evaluation and management of human bite wounds should follow the general principles outlined for animal bites, with irrigation and topical wound cleansing. Antimicrobials should be given as early as possible to all patients regardless of the appearance of the wound. A physician experienced in hand surgery should evaluate the wound to determine if the fascia is intact or if it has been penetrated. In rare instances, the force of a punch can sever a tendon or nerve or break a bone. These wounds, although often quite small, may extend deeply into the hand tissues, and relaxation of the fist may carry organisms into the deep compartments and potential spaces of the hand. Exploration under tourniquet control may be necessary. Clenched-fist injuries often require hospitalization and intravenous antimicrobial therapy with agents such as cefoxitin (1 g IV q6-8h), ampicillin/sulbactam (1.5 to 3 g IV q6h), ertapenem (1 g IV q24h). or some combination that covers *S aureus*, *Haemophilus* species, *Eikenella corrodens,* and β-lactamase-producing anaerobes (Table 5-1). *E corrodens* is usually resistant to first-generation cephalosporins (eg, cefazolin, cephalexin), macrolides (eg, erythromycin), clindamycin and aminoglycosides, and these agents should be avoided as monotherapy. In the type 1 β-lactam allergic patient, fluoroquinolones (eg, moxifloxacin, levofloxacin) plus clindamycin, or TMP/SMX plus metronidazole, may be useful. Ancillary measures include administration of tetanus toxoid as indicated. The duration of therapy is typically 4 weeks for septic arthritis and 6 weeks for osteomyelitis.

Other Infections
Potentially Transmitted by Bite Wounds

Risk factors for tetanus and the patient's prior immunization status against *Clostridium tetani* must be evaluated in the treatment of every bite wound injury. The Centers for Disease Control and Prevention (CDC) guidelines and protocols should be used to evaluate the adequacy of prior tetanus immunization (Table 5-4).

All cat, dog, and wild animal bite wounds should be evaluated for the potential transmission of rabies virus infection. The likelihood of the biting animal carrying the rabies virus should be evaluated on an individual basis depending on the genus and species of the biting animal and on local epidemiologic information about the potential transmission of the rabies virus. The CDC guidelines and protocols should be consulted to evaluate the need for rabies immunization based on the type of animal exposure. Table 5-5 contains detailed information regarding the rabies virus postexposure prophylaxis protocol.

Because monkeys are kept as pets, used in medical research, cared for in zoos, and encountered in the wild, their bites may be encountered more frequently in the medical-care setting than would be anticipated. Simian bite wound infections have a microbiologic picture similar to human bite wound infections, and antimicrobial therapy should include agents effective against *E corrodens*; complications such as osteomyelitis and flexion contractures of the hand are frequent. Of added significance is the transmission of *Herpes simae* (B-virus) by Old World (Macaca) monkeys. Therefore, information regarding the type of monkey implicated in a simian bite wound is critical in evaluating the need for prophylactic acyclovir treatment of such bite wounds.

Numerous other infectious diseases may be transmitted by animal bites. Brucellosis (*Brucella* species), blastomycosis (*Blastomyces dermatitidis*), tularemia (*Francisella tularensis*), cat scratch disease (*Bartonella henselae*), rat bite fever (*Streptobacillus moniliformis* and *Spirillum minus*),

Table 5-4: Tetanus Prophylaxis in Wound Management

History of Absorbed Tetanus Toxoid (Doses)	Clean, Minor Wounds		All Other Wounds*	
	*Td***	*TIG*	*Td***	*TIG*
Unknown or <3	Yes	No	Yes	Yes
≥3***	No†	No	No‡	No

*Such as, but not limited to, wounds contaminated with dirt, feces, soil, and saliva; puncture wounds; avulsions; and wounds resulting from missiles, crushing, burns and frostbite.

**For children <7 years old; DTP (DT, if pertussis vaccine is contraindicated) is preferred to tetanus toxoid alone. For persons >7 years of age, Td is preferred to tetanus toxoid alone.

***If only three doses of fluid toxoid have been received, then a fourth dose of toxoid, preferably an absorbed toxoid, should be given.

†Yes, if >10 years since last dose.

‡Yes, if >5 years since last dose. More frequent boosters are not needed and can accentuate side effects.

DT=diptheria and tetanus toxoids adsorbed for pediatric use; DTP=diptheria and tetanus toxoids and pertussis vaccine, adsorbed for pediatric use; Td=tetanus and diptheria toxoids adsorbed for adult use; TIG=tetanus immune globulin.

Adapted from Diphtheria, tetanus, and pertussis: recommendations for vaccine use and other preventive measures. Recommendations of the Immunization Practices Advisory committee (ACIP). *MMWR Recomm Rep* 1991;40:1-28.

bubonic plague (*Yersenia pestis*), leptospirosis (*Leptospira* species), erysipelothrix (*Erysipelothrix rhusiopathiae*), and seal finger (possible *Mycoplasma* species) are some of the other infections that can be transmitted by various domestic and wild animals.

Human bite wounds should be evaluated on an individual basis for the potential transmission of infectious agents other than the usual bacterial pathogens that cause bite wound infection. Hepatitis B virus, hepatitis C virus, human immunodeficiency virus (HIV), *Treponema pallidum*, and *Mycobacterium tuberculosis* can all be transmitted by bite wounds. The treating physician should ask the patient about the health and disease status of the assailant biter if such information is available.

Infections Associated With Trauma

Human skin has a natural elasticity that provides a significant degree of resistance to injurious forces. The basic structural components that account for this elasticity are the skin's fibroblast and elastin fibers. Skin can be stretched, compressed, and deformed in many ways, and will resume its natural shape after a short recovery. Occasionally, however, injurious forces will overcome the resistance to trauma and disrupt the skin. Infections may then occur.

How the injury or trauma occurs, as well as the location of the injuries, may provide clinicians with clues about the number and types of pathogens in the wound. Infecting micro-organisms may be derived from an exogenous source (ie, water borne from water-related injury or from the soil in soil-contaminated injury) or from the patient's endogenous microflora. Most infections that result from traumatic injury are associated with the common pyogenic pathogens *S aureus* or β-hemolytic *Streptococcus* (Table 5-6).

A significant difference exists in the types of organisms isolated from wound infections of the upper extremities (hands and arms) and those isolated from the lower extremities (legs and feet). *S aureus* and *S pyogenes* are

Table 5-5: Rabies Postexposure Prophylaxis Schedule

Vaccination Status	Treatment
Not previously vaccinated	Local wound cleansing
	Rabies-immune globulin (RIG)
	Vaccine

*These regimens are applicable for all age groups, including children.

**The deltoid area is the only acceptable site of vaccination for adults and older children. For younger children, the outer aspect of the thigh may be used. Vaccines should never be administered in the gluteal area.

predominant in upper extremity infections, whereas Enterobacteriaceae and *Bacteroides fragilis* are much more likely to be isolated from leg and feet infections.

Regimen*

All postexposure treatment should begin with immediate cleansing of all wounds with soap and water. If available, a virucidal agent, such as a povidone-iodine solution, should be used to irrigate the wounds.

For RIG, 20 IU/kg body weight. If anatomically feasible, the full dose should be infiltrated around the wounds and any remaining volume should be administered intra-muscularly (IM) at an anatomic site distant from vaccine administration. Also, RIG should not be administered in the same syringe as vaccine. Because RIG may partially suppress active production of antibody, no more than the recommended dose should be given.

Human diploid cell vaccine (HDCV), rabies vaccine adsorbed (RVA), or purified chick embryo cell vaccine (PCEC) 1 mL, IM into deltoid area,** one each on days 0, 3, 7, 14, and 28.

5

†Any person with a history of pre-exposure vaccination with HDCV, RVA, or PCEC; prior postexposure prophylaxis with HDCV, RVA, or PCEC; or previous vaccination with any other type of rabies vaccine and a documented history of a response to the prior vaccination.

Adapted from Human rabies prevention--United States, 1999. Recommendations of the Advisory Committee on Immunization Practices (ACIP). *MMWR Recomm Rep* 1999;48:1-21.

(continued on next page)

Specific infections are associated with certain conditions. *Erysipelothrix rhusiopathiae* can cause cutaneous infections of the fingers and hands of fishermen, butchers,

Table 5-5: Rabies Postexposure Prophylaxis Schedule (continued)

Vaccination Status	Treatment
Previously vaccinated[†]	Local wound cleansing
	RIG
	Vaccine

*These regimens are applicable for all age groups, including children.

**The deltoid area is the only acceptable site of vaccination for adults and older children. For younger children, the outer aspect of the thigh may be used. Vaccines should never be administered in the gluteal area.

or abattoir workers. Nail puncture wounds of the foot often are infected with *P aeruginosa*.

Specific infections associated with water immersion injuries include those caused by *Vibrio vulnificus*, *Aeromonas hydrophila*, *Plesiomonas shigelloides*, and *Chromobacterium* species. *V vulnificus* often causes spreading necrotizing infection in wounds that are contaminated in salt or brackish water (Figure 5-6, see color plate insert). Primary cutaneous infection usually follows injury occurring in seawater. Cutaneous penetration may occur via wounds that develop while in the water or as a result of exposure to pre-existing wounds. Wounds that are sustained during

Regimen*

All postexposure treatment should begin with immediate thorough cleaning of all wounds with soap and water. If available, a virucidal agent, such as a povidone-iodine solution, should be used to irrigate the wounds.

RIG should not be administered.

HDCV, RVA, or PCEC 1 mL, IM into deltoid area,** one each on days 0 and 3.

†Any person with a history of pre-exposure vaccination with HDCV, RVA, or PCEC; prior postexposure prophylaxis with HDCV, RVA, or PCEC; or previous vaccination with any other type of rabies vaccine and a documented history of a response to the prior vaccination.

Adapted from Human rabies prevention--United States, 1999. Recommendations of the Advisory Committee on Immunization Practices (ACIP). *MMWR Recomm Rep* 1999;48:1-21.

5

shellfish gathering (ie, cleaning crabs, peeling shrimp, shucking oysters) are also susceptible. Patients with underlying problems of alcoholism and cirrhosis are at the highest risk for developing systemic *V vulnificus* infection. Clinically, *V vulnificus* infection is usually characterized by an initial cellulitis, but the infection may be accompanied by bacteremia and shock. The cellulitis characteristically is associated with subcutaneous involvement and necrotizing hemorrhagic formation. This is often an extension to the subcutaneous tissues, including muscle. Seventy-five percent of patients have metastatic skin lesions, most commonly manifesting as bullous lesions. Wounds caused

Table 5-6: Bacteriology of Nonsurgical Wounds

Pathogen	Upper Extremity (hand, arm) N=75*	Lower Extremity (leg, feet) N=181*
Aerobes		
S aureus	34	46
S pyogenes	18	15
Enterococcus	0	15
Enterobacteriaceae	2	55
Pseudomonas sp	6	19
Other aerobes	40	34
Anaerobes		
Anaerobic gram-positive cocci	30	92
Clostridium sp	12	37
B fragilis	3	36
Other *Bacteroides* sp	35	34
Other anaerobes	31	20

*Number of patients

by freshwater immersion injuries may be infected with *A hydrophila*. In the normal host, this bacterium may produce a rapidly progressive cellulitis and soft-tissue infection. In compromised hosts, however, a more serious infection may occur, including bacteremia, central nervous system (CNS) infection, endocarditis, and peritonitis. *P shigelloides* can produce similar infections through contact with fresh water. *Chromobacterium violaceum* is a facultative gram-negative bacillus commonly found in the waters of tropical and semitropical regions, including the southeastern United States, which can also cause skin lesions.

Clinicians need to appreciate the implications of infections with these organisms to achieve appropriate management because these infections often are associated with rapid necrosis of skin that requires early, appropriate debridement. Such pathogens also typically are not susceptible to antimicrobial agents that might be used to treat staphylococcal or streptococcal infections (Table 5-1). *V vulnificus* is usually susceptible to the fluoroquinolones (ie, ciprofloxacin), aminoglycosides, and third-generation cephalosporins. *Plesiomonas* species and *Aeromonas* species are usually susceptible to the fluoroquinolones, ie, ceftazidime, cefepime; the carbapenems, ie, meropenem, imipenem/cilastatin; and the aminoglycosides.

Infections Associated With Pressure Ulcers

Secondary infections of pressure ulcers are common in elderly and immobile patients, and can be associated with severe morbidity and sepsis. Pressure ulcers are localized areas of tissue necrosis that develop in response to the tissue necrosis that occurs secondary to pressure, usually over a bony prominence. Subsequent wounds often are referred to as decubitus ulcers, bedsores, or pressure sores. Pressure ulcers represent a continuum from soft-tissue erythema to deep wounds extending through the fascia and into the muscle. Pressure ulcers can be classified into four categories (Table 5-7):

Stage I: Nonblanchable erythema of intact skin

Stage II: Partial thickness skin loss

Stage III: Full thickness skin loss

Stage IV: Deeper full thickness lesions extending into muscle or bone

Table 5-7: Pressure Ulcer Classification

Stage	Description
Stage I	Nonblanchable erythema of intact skin— the heralding lesion of pressure ulcers
Stage II	Partial thickness skin loss involving the epidermis or dermis
Stage III	Full thickness skin loss involving subcutaneous tissue that may extend to, but not through, the underlying fascia
Stage IV	Deeper, full-thickness lesions extending into muscle or bone

Source: The National Pressure Ulcer Advisory Panel

Estimates of the prevalence of pressure ulcers range from 3% to 14% among patients in acute care hospital settings, and from 15% to 25% among patients in skilled nursing facilities. Most patients with pressure ulcers are older than 70 years of age; a fourfold risk of death has been reported among geriatric patients with pressure ulcers. The most frequent sites of pressure ulcers, the coccyx-sacral area and heels, are particularly susceptible to colonization and secondary infection with mixed aerobic and anaerobic micro-organisms, which are derived from fecal flora (Figure 5-7 see color plate insert).

Immobility is the most important risk factor and contributing condition to the development of pressure ulcers, except in certain situations, as when an ulcer occurs beneath a cast. The underlying host factors are those that cause decreased movement, such as cerebrovascular diseases, spinal cord injury, rheumatologic disease, and musculoskeletal disease. Fecal incontinence increases the risk of infection of decubitus ulcers, which may progress to necrotizing skin infection and sepsis. Age-related changes in skin, including decreases in turgor and elasticity, also increase the susceptibility of skin to breakdown in the elderly.

Four factors have been implicated in the pathogenesis of skin breakdown: (1) pressure, (2) shearing forces, (3) friction, and (4) moisture. A short duration of pressure-induced ischemia is followed by reactive hyperemia. When this ischemia is prolonged, plasma leaks into the involved area, producing a bulbous lesion. Hemorrhage can occur and lead to nonblanchable erythema. In animals with bacteremia, bacteria are deposited at sites of pressure-induced ischemia and may cause suppurative lesions. The accumulation of toxic metabolites and the lack of nutrients resulting from occlusion of blood vessels in lymphatic channels may lead to necrosis of subcutaneous tissue and muscle and, ultimately, of the dermis and epidermis. Pressure may cause the formation of subepidermal blisters. Pressure is most prominent under bony prominences, such as the sacrum and greater trochanter in patients confined to bedrest. Shearing forces are generated when a seated person slides toward the floor, or when a recumbent person slides toward the foot of the bed when the head of the bed is elevated. In these situations, sacral skin is stationary in relation to the support service, whereas the subcutaneous tissue and deep gluteal vessels are stretched and angulated. Frictional forces, such as those generated by pulling a patient across a bedsheet, may cause intraepidermal blisters and, ultimately, superficial erosions. Moisture can increase the friction between two surfaces and may lead to maceration and eventually superficial skin breakdown.

Available data suggest that older people and persons with spinal cord injuries are at the highest risk for developing pressure ulcers. Risk factors associated with pressure ulcers include immobility, hypoalbuminemia, the presence of a frac-

Table 5-8: Bacteriology of Pressure (Decubitus) Ulcers

Pathogen	Galpin et al N=21**	Bryan et al N=62	Brook* N=58
Group A Streptococcus (GAS)	2	3	9
Enterococcus	11	2	4
Other Streptococcus	1	6	8
S aureus	6	10	25
Coagulase-negative Staphylococcus	5	3	5
Other aerobes	3	0	28
Enterobacteriaceae	33	25[1]	17
Pseudomonas sp	5	3	7
Bacteroides sp	5	10	15
Clostridium sp	3	0	2
Other anaerobes	4	0	36

*Children
**Number of patients
[1] 12 of 25 were Proteus mirabilis

ture, fecal incontinence (but not urinary incontinence), urinary catheter use, diarrhea, increased age, dementia, poor health, dry or scaling skin, cigarette smoking, and inactivity.

Pressure ulcers are associated with potentially serious infectious complications. Mortality approaches 50% in hospitalized patients with sepsis associated with pressure ulcers. Outbreaks of nosocomial infection have been associated with bacterial colonization and clinical infection of pressure ulcers.

The bacteriology of clinically infected pressure ulcers, particularly those in the sacral, perineal, or lower extremity areas, usually includes mixed polymicrobial pathogens (Table 5-8). Patients from long-term care facilities who have decubitus ulcers may constitute an important reservoir for the spread of MRSA.

The outcome of pressure ulcer infections depends on the underlying focal and systemic conditions, as well as on the extent of the lesion. Avoidance of further pressure, relief of edema, and good nutrition are hallmarks for proper care of chronic pressure ulcers. Antimicrobial therapy should be considered only when intense local inflammatory reaction or systemic symptoms are present. Hospitalization is not necessary when the lesion is localized. Local care includes relief of pressure, debridement followed by wet-to-dry dressing changes, improvement of host nutrition, relief of edema by elevation and diuretic therapy, and improvement of vascular supply when applicable. Topical agents that are promoted commercially or through anecdotal reports should be viewed cautiously because most of these agents have not been tested under double-blind conditions. The potential for underlying deeper infections (ie, osteomyelitis, tendon involvement, deep abscess), should be investigated. As with other open wound and sinus tract infections, interpretation of the results of superficial wound culture is difficult, but operative culture should be obtained before committing to definitive long-term treatment. Selected antimicrobial agents (ie, β-lactam/β-lactamase inhibitor combinations, imipenem) should have a spectrum of activity that includes aerobic and anaerobic flora and, specifically, *S aureus*.

Infected Cysts and Abscesses

Epidermal cysts can become secondarily infected with subsequent abscess formation. The dominant causative

Table 5-9: Organisms Isolated From Epidermal Cysts

Pathogens	Head N=41	Neck N=24
Aerobes only (%)	20	54
Anaerobes only (%)	44	33
Aerobes and anaerobes (%)	27	13

Predominant Organisms (N)

Aerobes

	Head	Neck
β-hemolytic *Streptococcus*	4	5
Other *Streptococcus*	4	1
S aureus	16	11
Enterobacteriaceae	—	1
Pseudomonas	—	—
Eikenella	2	—

Anaerobes

	Head	Neck
Gram-positive cocci	21	9
Propionibacterium	3	2
Clostridium	—	—
Fusobacterium	—	—
Prevotella sp	4	1
Bacteroides sp	12	6

From Brook I, *Arch Dermatol* 1989;125:1658-1661.

Trunk N=31	Extremities N=56	Rectal N=27
55	68	7
29	14	26
16	18	67
—	3	1
6	5	2
13	34	6
1	2	10
—	2	3
—	2	—
16	19	12
1	1	—
—	—	1
1	—	—
1	—	2
3	—	23

organisms are *S aureus* and aerobic streptococci (Table 5-9). Although *S aureus* is the predominant isolate, especially in trunk and extremity infections, anaerobes are frequently isolated in cyst abscesses in rectal areas. Polymicrobial abscesses are also common close to the oral cavity. These anaerobes include *Prevotella*, *Fusobacterium*, and *Peptostreptococcus* species around the mouth, and *B fragilis*, *Peptostreptococcus*, and *Clostridium* species around the anal area (Enterobacteriaceae may also be found there). Management includes surgical drainage and antimicrobial therapy (Table 5-1).

Perianal cysts and abscesses occur commonly from anal crypts, from which infection spreads through muscle to create an anal fistula. Pilonidal cysts are seen most commonly in young men with hirsutism and intertrigo as predisposing conditions. Pilonidal sinuses are formed by hair shafts ingrowing into skin of the natal cleft; an inflammatory reaction leads to formation of a squamous epithelial-lined pit. Secondary infections may occur, resulting in abscess tracks.

Surgical drainage is the therapy of choice for an epidermal cyst abscess. This is particularly important because the environment of an abscess is detrimental for many antimicrobials. The abscess capsule, the low pH, and the presence of inactivating enzymes (ie, β-lactamases) may impair the activity of many antimicrobials. Because of these limitations, drainage is still the therapy of choice for an abscess. However, administration of systemic antimicrobials is indicated in selected cases, such as in immunocompromised patients or in instances in which local or systemic spread of the infection has occurred. Management of mixed infections caused by aerobic and anaerobic bacteria requires the administration of antimicrobials effective against both aerobic and anaerobic components of the infection. Antimicrobials that provide coverage for *S aureus*, as well as anaerobic bacteria, include cefoxitin, cefotetan, imipenem/cilastatin, meropenem, ampicillin/sulbactam, piperacillin/tazobactam, ticarcillin/clavulanate, and the combination of clindamycin and a fluoroquinolone.

Treatment should be guided by culture results. Surgical excision should be considered for patients who experience frequent recurrences.

Selected Readings

Baddour LM, Bisno AL: Recurrent cellulitis after saphenous venectomy for coronary bypass surgery. *Ann Intern Med* 1982;97:493-496.

Bratzler DW: The Surgical Infection Prevention and Surgical Care Improvement Projects: promises and pitfalls. *Am Surg* 2006;72: 1010-1016.

Brook I: Cellulitis and fasciitis. *Current Treatment Options in Infectious Diseases* 2000;2:127-146.

Brook I: Microbiological studies of decubitus ulcers in children. *J Pediatr Surg* 1991;26:207-209.

Brook I: Microbiology of human and animal bite wounds in children. *Pediatr Infect Dis J* 1987;6:29-32.

Brook I: Microbiology of infected epidermal cysts. *Arch Dermatol* 1989;125:1658-1661.

Brook I, Frazier EH: Aerobic and anaerobic bacteriology of chronic venous ulcers. *Int J Dermatol* 1998;37:426-428.

Brook I, Frazier EH: Aerobic and anaerobic bacteriology of wounds and cutaneous abscesses. *Arch Surg* 1990;125:1445-1451.

Bryan CS, Dew CE, Reynolds KL: Bacteremia associated with decubitus ulcers. *Arch Intern Med* 1983;143:2093-2095.

Chuang YC, Yuan CY, Liu CY, et al: *Vibrio vulnificus* infection in Taiwan: report of 28 cases and review of clinical manifestations and treatment. *Clin Infect Dis* 1992;15:271-276.

File TM Jr, Tan JS: Treatment of bacterial skin and soft tissue infections. *Surg Gynecol Obstet* 1991;172(suppl):17-24.

Galpin JE, Chow AW, Bayer AS, et al: Sepsis associated with decubitus ulcers. *Am J Med* 1976;61:346-350.

Gold WL, Salit IE: *Aeromonas hydrophila* infections of skin and soft tissue: report of 11 cases and review. *Clin Infect Dis* 1993;16:69-74.

Goldstein EJ: Bite wounds. *Current Treatment Options in Infectious Diseases* 2000;2:173-180.

Goldstein EJ: New horizons in bacteriology, antimicrobial susceptibility and therapy of animal bite wounds. *J Med Microbiol* 1998;47:95-97.

5

Mangram AJ, Horan TC, Pearson MI, et al: Guideline for prevention of surgical site infection, 1999. Hospital Infection Control Practices Advisory Committee. *Infect Control Hosp Epidemiol* 1999;20:250-278.

National Nosocomial Infections Surveillance (NNIS) System report, data summary from January 1990-May 1999, issued June 1999. *Am J Infect Control* 1999;27:520-532.

Patel CV, Powell L, Wilson SE: Surgical wound infections. *Current Treatment Options in Infectious Diseases* 2000;2:147-153.

Pressure ulcers prevalence, cost and risk assessment: consensus development conference statement. The National Pressure Ulcer Advisory Panel. *Decubitus* 1989;2:24-33.

Sherertz RJ, Garibaldi RA, Marosok RD, et al: Consensus paper on the surveillance of surgical wound infections. *Am J Infect Control* 1992;20:263-270.

Stevens DL, Bisno AL, Chambers HF, et al, and the Infectious Diseases Society of America: Practice guidelines for the diagnosis and management of skin and soft-tissue infections. *Clin Infect Dis* 2005;41:1373-1406.

Stevens DL: Cellulitis, pyoderma, abscesses and other skin and subcutaneous infections. In: Cohen J, Powderly WG, et al, eds: *Infectious Diseases,* 2nd ed. Edinburgh, Scotland, Mosby, 2003, pp 133-144.

Swartz MN, Pasternack MS: Cellulitis and subcutaneous tissue infections. In: Mandell Gl, Bennett JE, Dolin R, eds: *Principles and Practice of Infectious Diseases*, 6th ed. New York, NY, Churchill Livingstone, 2005, pp 1172-1193.

Swartz MN: Cellulitis and subcutaneous tissue infections. In: Mandell GL, Bennett JE, Dolin R, eds: *Principles and Practice of Infectious Diseases*, 5th ed. New York, NY, Churchill Livingstone, 2000, pp 1037-1057.

Talan DA, Citron DM, Abrahamian FM, et al: Bacteriologic analysis of infected dog and cat bites. Emergency Medicine Animal Bite Infection Study Group. *N Engl J Med* 1999;340:85-92.

Talan DA, Abrahamian FM, Moran GJ, et al, and the Emergency Medicine Human Bite Infection Study Group. Clinical presentation and bacteriologic analysis of infected human bites in patients presenting to emergency departments. *Clin Infect Dis* 2003;37:1481-1489.

Tan JS: Human zoonotic infections transmitted by dogs and cats. *Arch Intern Med* 1997;157:1933-1943.

Chapter 6

Common Diabetic Foot Infections and Their Complications

D iabetic patients are prone to infectious complications. In these patients, foot infections are the most common complication and are responsible for more days of hospitalization than any other complication. Diabetes is also the leading cause of lower extremity amputation. In fact, the rate of lower extremity amputation in diabetics is estimated to be as much as 40 times greater than in nondiabetics. Of those patients who require extremity amputations, 9 of 10 will be insulin dependent. This chapter reviews management of diabetic patients with foot infections, with an emphasis on the importance of early recognition of foot problems through clinical examination and appropriate laboratory diagnosis. We will also examine the roles of timely surgical and medical interventions.

6

Pathophysiology

The diabetic patient's susceptibility to foot infection is caused by three metabolic abnormalities associated with the disease—neuropathy, vasculopathy, and immunopathy. These abnormalities are highly prevalent in diabetic patients.

Among diabetic patients, neuropathy predisposes the foot to trauma and infections, while angiopathy influences the outcome. Neuropathy is responsible for the breakdown of the patient's first line of defense, the intact skin. Autonomic neuropathy reduces moisture to the skin and predisposes it to crack. The foot with sensory neuropathy tends to be injured repeatedly, disrupting skin integrity and providing a point of entry for bacteria. Motor neuropathy results in atrophic changes of the intrinsic foot muscles, altering the foot architecture and changing the pressure points of the involved foot (Figure 6-1, see color plate insert). This change predisposes the foot to repeated pressure injuries because the foot strikes the ground during ambulation.

Vasculopathy may result in both macro- and microangiopathy. The vascular disease process, in conjunction with autonomic vasomotor impairment, may cause local hypoxia, atrophy, and necrosis. The combination of neuropathy and vasculopathy may also accelerate the process of soft-tissue breakdown. Deficient circulation may retard wound healing, and open wounds invite infection. Immunopathy manifests in several ways. Metabolic abnormalities have been implicated in defects in polymorphonuclear leukocyte function (ie, adherence, chemotaxis, phagocytosis, microbial killing). Poor wound healing, defective granuloma formation, and prolonged persistence of abscesses have been described in animals rendered experimentally diabetic.

The loss of skin integrity from trauma, fungal infection of the interdigital web spaces, paronychia, or puncture wounds is a major predisposing factor. Other risk factors for infection and subsequent amputation include nonhealing foot ulcers, infection, advanced age, male sex, black race, and a history of smoking. Wound healing depends on adequate blood supply, which is commonly impaired among diabetic patients.

Classification

The medical literature includes numerous classifications of diabetic foot infections. A practical clinical approach is presented in the Infectious Diseases Society of America (IDSA) Diabetic Foot Guidelines (Table 6-1), which groups foot infections as mild, moderate (potentially limb threatening), and severe (potentially life threatening). An uninfected wound lacks purulence or any manifestations of inflammation. This is an important point because it is clear that the diagnosis of infection in these ulcerations should be made on a clinical basis. Microbiologic testing of such lesions will lead to a false-positive result because many colonizing bacteria will invariably grow from a swab culture. This may lead to the mistaken conclusion that these are infected lesions that need antibiotic treatment. Using antibiotics in clinically uninfected wounds adds no benefit over standard therapy without antibiotics. Theoretically, in addition to other adverse drug effects, using inappropriate antibiotics in clinically uninfected wounds could lead to resistance. Clinically uninfected wounds should be managed with local wound care including debridement, dressings, and offloading.

A wound with a mild infection presents with purulence or <2 manifestations of inflammation including erythema, pain, tenderness, warmth, or induration. The cellulitis must be localized extending ≤2 cm around the ulcer. These are superficial infections with no systemic complications. Commonly encountered superficial infections include paronychia, infected ingrown toenail, infected shallow ulcer on the plantar surface (Figure 6-2, see color plate insert), and web-space infection between the toes. Web-space infections caused by either dermatophytes or erythrasma frequently are unnoticed because the patient or the caregiver fails to perform routine inspections of the feet. These infections provide a nidus for bacteria growth that may lead to a deep-space abscess or cellulitis. Deep-foot infections may also be preceded by paronychia, infected toenail, or superficial ulcerations.

A moderate infection is one in which the patient is both systemically well and metabolically stable, but also has more than one of the following characteristics—cellulitis spreading beyond 2 cm around the ulcer, streaking, a deep-tissue abscess, gangrene, or deep-tissue spread.

Table 6-1: Classification of Foot Ulcers Based on Clinical Severity

Clinical Severity	Characteristics
Mild	Presence of ≥2 manifestations of inflammation (purulence or erythema, pain, tenderness, warmth, or induration), but any cellulitis/erythema that extends ≤2 cm around ulcer and infection is limited to the skin or superficial subcutaneous tissues. No other local complications or systemic illness is present.
Moderate to severe (potentially limb threatening)	• Ulceration to deep tissues • Purulent discharge • Cellulitis • Systemic toxicity • Mild-to-moderate necrosis • Presence/absence of osteomyelitis
Severe (potentially life threatening)	• Ulceration to deep tissues • Purulent discharge • Cellulitis • Systemic toxicity, including septic shock • Marked necrosis/gangrene • Presence/absence of osteomyelitis • Bacteremia

Therapy
- Oral antibiotics
- Local podiatry care

- Intravenous antibiotics
- Surgical drainage/excision of deep sepsis
- Prolonged antibiotic therapy and/or
  bone resection for osteomyelitis
- Assess need for revascularization

- Urgent surgical debridement, drainage,
  or amputation
- Intravenous broad-spectrum antibiotics
- Control hyperglycemia and ketoacidosis
- Assess need for revascularization

From: Grayson, *Infect Dis Clin North Am* 1995;9:143-161.

Finally, a severe infection presents with all of the clinical findings in the moderate category but in a patient who is metabolically unstable, systemically unwell, or with significant peripheral arterial disease. Often such infections involve the deep soft tissues of the foot. Deep-foot infections are divided into three types—dorsal foot phlegmon, deep plantar space infections, and infected foot ulcers. If left unattended, any of these deep-foot infections may result in osteomyelitis, limb loss, sepsis, and even death. Dorsal foot phlegmon, or cellulitis, usually begins as an infection at the base of the toenail or in the web space. Subsequently, it spreads to the rest of the foot. It is commonly seen as a swollen erythematous lesion involving the base of the involved toe and spreads to the distal third of the foot. This swelling may extend beyond the ankle. Systemic symptoms (ie, fever, chills, malaise) are common. The presence of skin necrosis implies impaired arterial supply. Deep plantar space infections of the foot frequently originate from web-space infection, nail-bed infection, and, less commonly, from direct puncture. The medial, lateral, and central plantar spaces are usually affected (Figures 6-3a and 6-3b, see color plate inserts). Infections of the medial and lateral spaces do not threaten any important deep tissue other than the adjacent bone. Prognosis is usually good, if treated early. On the other hand, infection of the central plantar space is the most serious, and frequently requires surgical intervention. Patients with central space infection have a red, swollen foot, and frequently present with fever, chills, malaise, and hyperglycemia. Pus may fill this space, resulting in the loss of skin creases and the foot's longitudinal arch. Swelling may occur behind the medial malleolus because of its connection to the central plantar space. Complications from central space infection include toe gangrene from compromised arterial blood flow at the arch or the digital branches, ischemic necrosis of intrinsic foot muscles, suppurative tendonitis, arthritis, and even sepsis. When the infection spreads beyond the central plantar space, destruction of the interosseous fascia permits micro-organisms to directly invade the dorsum of the foot, and to extend along the flexor tendons to the calf and lower leg regions.

A foot infection is considered mild or nonlimb threatening when the ulceration is superficial (Figure 6-2, see color plate insert), purulent discharge is not seen on examination, cellulitis is minimal or absent, and systemic toxicity is not found. Moderate-to-severe or potentially limb-threatening infection occurs when the ulceration extends to the deeper tissues (Figure 6-4, see color plate insert), when purulence is noted, cellulitis is present, systemic toxicity is detected, or mild-to-moderate necrosis is observed. The presence of osteomyelitis is an indication of deep infection but not an important finding for classification of severity. Severe or potentially life-threatening infection occurs when the patient has systemic toxicity with or without septic shock, the foot shows marked necrosis or gangrene, or bacteremia is detected.

Diagnosis

Early recognition of foot infection in a diabetic patient is critical. Unfortunately, most practicing physicians do not routinely examine the feet of a diabetic patient during an office visit, nor do they adequately instruct their patients to do daily foot inspections. A detailed neurologic examination of the feet is mandatory to detect sensory, motor, or autonomic neuropathy. Numbness, loss of sensation, lack of sweating, decreased ankle jerk, flattened plantar arch, dorsiflexion hammer toe, splaying of toes, and Charcot's foot are common manifestations. The best method to detect sensory neuropathy is the use of a monofilament. Normally, the patient should be able to feel pressure from the monofilament when it is applied to the point of buckling (Figure 6-5, see color plate insert). In advanced cases, the patient does not feel pressure applied to the Achilles tendon. If foot architecture deformity is suspected, a radiographic examination of the feet should be taken to look for neuropathic changes, fractures, and/or osteomyelitis. When signs of vascular insufficiency are present, further studies should be undertaken to determine the need for augmentation of vascular supply.

The physician must look for manifestations of angiopathy, such as claudication, cold feet, resting pain, dependent rubor (ie, redness developing after the foot is placed in a dependent position), diminished pulse, decreased leg blood pressure (less than the arm), blanching on elevation, delayed venous filling, shiny skin, atrophic subcutaneous tissue, or thickened nails.

Regardless of its depth, a foot ulcer should alert the clinician to search for deep-tissue infection, such as osteomyelitis. We recommend applying a metal probe to the ulcer. When the probe can reach the bone, the positive predictive value for osteomyelitis is close to 90%. Foot radiograph is helpful in the diagnosis of osteomyelitis, but a negative finding does not rule out infection.

Microbiologic diagnosis is important because diabetic patients may need antimicrobial therapy. Inappropriate cultures are commonly taken by inexperienced personnel. Swabbing a superficial wound for culture has been shown to yield unreliable results. A low concordance has been shown between cultures of a superficial wound and cultures of a deep-tissue lesion. A needle or open biopsy of the infected site should provide a more reliable result. Knowing the etiologic agent or agents that cause a wound infection is generally helpful in selecting definitive antibiotic therapy. Obtain specimens for culture before initiating antibiotic therapy, if possible, or after discontinuing it (in a stable patient who has failed to respond) for a few days. To avoid identifying contaminants, obtain and process specimens using appropriate methods. Tissue samples from a debrided wound generally provide more accurate culture results than superficial swabs. Most studies indicate that the latter yield a greater range of organisms than deeper material, and yet may still fail to identify some of the deep flora.

Table 6-2: Obtaining Soft-Tissue Cultures From a Diabetic Foot Infection

When

- Culturing clinically uninfected lesions is unnecessary, unless done as part of an infection control surveillance protocol.

- Cultures of infected wounds are valuable in directing antibiotic choices, but may be unnecessary with an acute mild infection in an antibiotic-naive patient.

- Blood cultures should be obtained from patients with a severe infection, especially if they are systemically ill.

How

- Cleanse and debride the lesion before obtaining specimens for culture.

- With an open wound, obtain tissue from the debrided base, whenever possible, by curettage (scraping with a sterile dermal curette or scalpel blade) or biopsy (bedside or operative).

- Avoid swabs of undebrided ulcers or wound drainage. If swabbing the debrided wound base is the only available culture option, use a swab designed for culturing aerobic and anaerobic organisms and rapidly transport it to the laboratory.

- Needle aspiration may be useful for obtaining purulent collections, or perhaps a specimen from an area of cellulitis.

- Clearly identify samples (eg, specimen type, anatomic location) and promptly send them to the laboratory in an appropriate sterile container or transport media for aerobic and anaerobic cultures.

From: Infectious Diseases Society of America (IDSA) Guidelines on the Management of Diabetic Foot Infections

Standard swab specimens yield fewer anaerobes and are often minimally processed by the microbiology laboratory, but, properly collected and transported, anaerobic swab specimens may be adequate. Skin aspiration may yield a pathogen in cases of cellulitis, but this method is insensitive and the pathogens in these cases are predictably aerobic gram-positive cocci. Table 6-2 describes how to obtain soft-tissue cultures from a diabetic foot infection.

Blood cultures should be obtained in those who are hospitalized. Anaerobic bacteria may be isolated from the blood cultures and not from the infected site. For osteomyelitis in diabetic patients, it is helpful to obtain samples from both the bone and the overlying infected tissues. Table 6-3 lists the various imaging techniques to diagnose osteomyelitis.

Plain radiographic study of the foot is the most cost-effective imaging study. It can detect gas in the tissues, long-standing osteomyelitis, or neuropathic bone changes, but it lacks sensitivity in detecting early osteomyelitis. Cortical bone disruption is a radiographic sign for osteomyelitis. Technetium bone scan is not recommended as a screening test because it is expensive and not specific in diagnosing osteomyelitis. Positive scans are also found in patients with fracture and gout. The indium-labeled leukocyte scan has been shown to be more specific. In a small study, Tc 99m HMPAO leukocyte scan showed strong potential. Dual-isotope scanning, which combines bone scan and indium-labeled leukocyte scan, provides higher sensitivity and specificity. Radioisotopic imaging is useful but expensive and should be restricted to cases when it can affect surgical treatment decisions. Magnetic resonance imaging (MRI) has been shown to be sensitive and specific, but not consistently by all investigators.

Probing to bone, in concert with radiographic and clinical evaluation, may be the most cost-effective diagnostic test for osteomyelitis before surgical debridement and definitive bone biopsy.

Table 6-3: Diagnosis of Osteomyelitis Using Different Diagnostic Imaging Techniques

Diagnostic Test	Number of Patients Studied	Sensitivity (%)	Specificity (%)
Dual-isotope scans (Tc 99m MDP bone scan *plus* in-labeled leukocyte scans)	31	93	83
MRI	22	91	77
Plain radiograph	27	22	94
Tc-bone scan	22	50	50
Indium-labeled leukocyte scan	19	33	69
MRI (19 patients had all four tests)	27	88	100
Radiograph, plain	77	69	82
Three-phase bone scan		100	38
Indium 111-labeled leukocyte scan		100	78
Bone scan *plus* leukocyte scan		100	79
Radiograph, plain	20	73	40
MRI		77	40
Three-phase bone scan *plus* Indium 111-labeled leukocyte scan		63	100
Radiograph, plain	27	55	57
Three-phase bone scan		75	29
Tc 99m HMPAO leukocyte scan		90	86

MRI=magnetic resonance imaging
Modified from Lipsky (1997).

Treatment

The primary objective in the management of diabetic patients with foot infection is to return the foot to a functional capacity. Figure 6-6 is an algorithm that shows the proper care of a patient with suspected diabetic foot infection. Every effort should be made to remove necrotic and infected tissue. This results in better control of infection and more rapid healing. A team approach to care of these patients is beneficial and cost effective. The team should consist of the primary care physician, endocrinologist, infectious disease expert, and a surgeon with expertise in the care of foot and ankle diseases.

The roles of the primary care physician and the endocrinologist are to ensure proper patient education about foot care and to maintain good glycemic control. The role of the infectious disease expert is to manage the infection by choosing reasonable empiric antimicrobial therapy, collecting proper specimens for microbiology, implementing appropriate selection of final antimicrobial therapy, and determining the duration of treatment. The surgeon's involvement should start as early as possible. The decision for aggressive and timely debridement, amputation, and revascularization rests on his or her experience and skill.

Surgical intervention is often necessary to control diabetic foot infections. A decision may have to be made about the need for ablative surgery. Infected ulcers may have to be debrided thoroughly. Early incision and drainage decreases the inoculum size of infecting micro-organisms and may accelerate local healing. Before definitive surgery, a trial of appropriate antimicrobial therapy may be indicated to maximize control of cellulitis and to minimize the extent of infection at the intended surgical site. As much of the limb as is necessary must be preserved for future rehabilitation and ambulation, but not so much as to compromise control of the infectious state. Localized osteomyelitis often requires limited surgical ablation, such as toe amputation, ray resection, transmetatarsal amputation, or through-the-ankle (Syme's) amputation.

Removal of the infected bone decreases the duration of antimicrobial therapy, hastens recovery, and decreases the incidence of relapse. Recent studies have shown that early and limited surgical intervention with aggressive antimicrobial therapy may reduce the number of days of hospitalization, the incidence of relapse, and the need for above-ankle amputation in cases of diabetic foot infection.

In diabetic patients with deep infection of the foot, timely surgical intervention results in better outcome and reduction of limb loss (Figures 6-4a through 6-4d, see color plate insert). In our center, we compared early aggressive surgical approach combined with broad-spectrum antimicrobial therapy to broad-spectrum antimicrobial therapy alone with or without delayed surgical intervention after 72 hours (Figure 6-7). The rate of above-ankle amputation among our patients with infected foot was significantly reduced when early debridement or limited amputation with appropriate antimicrobial therapy was performed within the first 72 hours of hospital admission. Other investigators have also shown that early diagnosis and treatment, including surgical intervention of nongangrenous limb infections, reduced the need for amputation, thus reducing the total medical cost. Another aspect of care is the evaluation and intervention of arterial insufficiency. Augmentation of arterial supply is important in promoting better healing of foot lesions.

In some cases, amputation is the best or only option. Urgent amputation is usually required when there is extensive necrosis or life-threatening infection. Elective amputation may be considered in the patient with recurrent ulceration despite maximal preventive measures, with irreversible loss of foot function, or who would require unacceptably prolonged or intensive hospital care. Selecting the level of amputation must take into consideration vascular, reconstructive, and rehabilitation issues. A higher level amputation that results in a more functional residual stump (even if a prosthesis is required) may be a better choice than preserving a foot that is mechanically unsound, unlikely

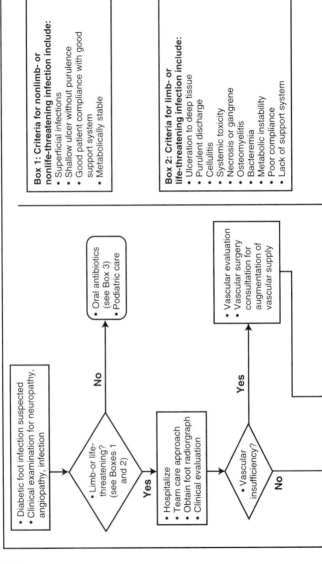

Box 1: Criteria for nonlimb- or nonlife-threatening infection include:
- Superficial infections
- Shallow ulcer without purulence
- Good patient compliance with good support system
- Metabolically stable

Box 2: Criteria for limb- or life-threatening infection include:
- Ulceration to deep tissue
- Purulent discharge
- Cellulitis
- Systemic toxicity
- Necrosis or gangrene
- Osteomyelitis
- Bacteremia
- Metabolic instability
- Poor compliance
- Lack of support system

- Diabetic foot infection suspected
- Clinical examination for neuropathy, angiopathy, infection

• Limb- or life-threatening? (see Boxes 1 and 2)

No
- Oral antibiotics (see Box 3)
- Podiatric care

Yes
- Hospitalize
- Team care approach
- Obtain foot radiograph
- Clinical evaluation

• Vascular insufficiency?

Yes
- Vascular evaluation
- Vascular surgery consultation for augmentation of vascular supply

No

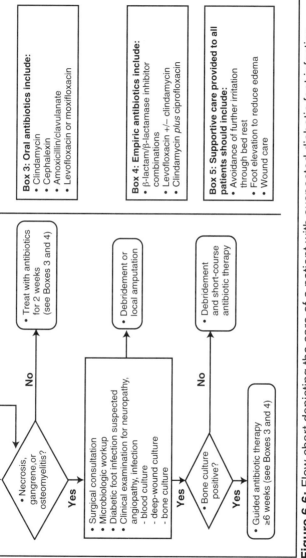

Box 3: Oral antibiotics include:
- Clindamycin
- Cephalexin
- Amoxicillin/clavulanate
- Levofloxacin or moxifloxacin

Box 4: Empiric antibiotics include:
- β-lactam/β-lactamase inhibitor combinations
- Levofloxacin +/− clindamycin
- Clindamycin *plus* ciprofloxacin

Box 5: Supportive care provided to all patients should include:
- Avoidance of further irritation through bed rest
- Foot elevation to reduce edema
- Wound care

- Necrosis, gangrene, or osteomyelitis?

No → Treat with antibiotics for 2 weeks (see Boxes 3 and 4)

Yes ↓

- Surgical consultation
- Microbiologic workup
- Diabetic foot infection suspected
- Clinical examination for neuropathy, angiopathy, infection
  - blood culture
  - deep-wound culture
  - bone culture

→ Debridement or local amputation

- Bone culture positive?

No → Debridement and short-course antibiotic therapy

Yes ↓

- Guided antibiotic therapy ≥6 weeks (see Boxes 3 and 4)

6

Figure 6-6: Flow chart depicting the care of a patient with suspected diabetic foot infection.

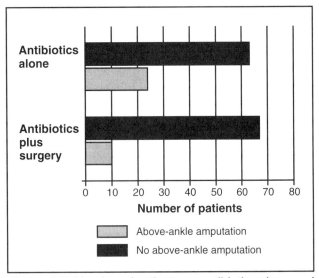

Figure 6-7: Number of patients on antibiotics alone and antibiotics plus early surgical intervention who did or did not have above-ankle amputation.

to heal, or could be prone to future ulceration. When all or part of a foot has dry gangrene, it may be preferable (especially in a patient who is a poor operative candidate) to let the necrotic portions auto-amputate. It may also be best to leave adherent eschar in place, especially on the heel, until it softens enough to be more easily removed, provided there does not appear to be an underlying focus of infection.

Choosing an Antibiotic Regimen

Antimicrobial therapy is usually begun before the availability of culture results. The choice of antimicrobial agents is based on an educated guess by the clinician. For example, most mild, superficial infections are caused by staphylococci and streptococci, so empiric oral therapy using antimicrobial agents with activity against these agents should be adequate. For patients with deeper infections, an antimicrobial agent that has both aerobic and anaerobic activity is recommended. Table 6-4 lists the recommended antimicrobial agents for empiric therapy.

Moderate-to-severe infections of the diabetic foot may require coverage of a broader spectrum of potential pathogens. Recently, emphasis has been given to the use of cost-effective, single-drug regimens that provide broad-spectrum coverage. Antimicrobial agents for these regimens include ertapenem (Invanz®), ampicillin/sulbactam (Unasyn®), ticarcillin/clavulanate (Timentin®), and piperacillin/tazobactam (Zosyn®IV). Another possible option, especially in a β-lactam allergic patient, is moxifloxacin (Avelox®), which has a broad spectrum of antimicrobial coverage (including anaerobes) and can be given on an oral once-daily basis. Although no studies have specifically addressed the efficacy of moxifloxacin in the treatment of the infected diabetic foot, the drug is indicated for complicated skin and skin-structure infections, and there are in vitro and clinical trials that suggest that it should be an effective antibiotic. In addition, tigecycline (Tygacil®) has broad-spectrum activity that includes *S aureus* (including methicillin-resistant *S aureus* [MRSA]), enterococcus, streptococcus spp., *Enterobacteriaciae*, and anaerobes (inactive for *Pseudomonas*). All of these drugs have a broad spectrum of activity that includes not only the aerobic gram-positive cocci, but also many gram-negative rods and anaerobic pathogens. As of this writing, ertapenem and piperacillin/tazobactam are the only drugs of this type to carry specific US Food and Drug Administration (FDA) indications for use in diabetic foot infections. Lipsky et al (2005) specifically studied ertapenem vs piperacillin/tazobactam in 445 infected diabetic feet, which is still the largest study to date in moderate-to-severe diabetic foot infections. The study demonstrated that ertapenem 1 g/day was at least as effective as piperacillin/tazobactam 3.375 g every 6 hours for the first 5 days, after which patients were given

6

Table 6-4: Suggested Empiric Therapy for Patients With Diabetic Foot Infections

Superficial Bacterial Infection (staphylococci and streptococci)

- <u>Penicillins:</u> dicloxacillin (Dynapen®), amoxicillin/clavulanate (Augmentin®, Augmentin®XR)

- <u>Oral cephalosporins:</u> cephalexin (Keflex®), cefadroxil (Duricef®, Ultracef®)

- <u>Allergic to penicillin:</u> clindamycin (Cleocin®) *plus* fluoroquinolones

- Methicillin-resistant *Staphylococcus aureus* (MRSA): If mild, can consider trimethoprim/sulfamethoxazole (TMP/SMX) (Bactrim™, Septra®) or clindamycin (if there is no inducible resistance reported by the microbiology laboratory) or oral linezolid (Zyvox®)

---

oral amoxicillin/clavulanate (Augmentin®, Augmentin® XR) 875/125 mg every 12 hours. Based on this study, the FDA granted ertapenem a specific indication for diabetic foot infections without osteomyelitis.

When confronted with a diabetic foot infection of any severity grade, the role of MRSA must be considered. As in many types of infection, both community-acquired (CA-MRSA) and hospital-acquired (HA-MRSA) strains have become more prevalent in the past few years. Daptomycin

Deep Bacterial Infection
(mixed aerobic/anaerobic bacteria)

- β-lactam/β-lactamase inhibitor combinations:
  ampicillin/sulbactam (Unasyn®),
  ticarcillin/clavulanate (Timentin®),
  piperacillin/tazobactam (Zosyn®IV)

- cefoxitin (Mefoxin®)

- ertapenem (Invanz®)

- imipenem/cilastatin (Primaxin®)

- meropenem (Merrem®, Merrem®IV)

- tigecycline (Tygacil®)

- clindamycin *plus* a fluoroquinolone
  (ie, ciprofloxacin [Cipro®],
  levofloxacin [Levaquin®])

- trovafloxacin (reserved for life-threatening or
  limb-threatening infections in the hospital)

- MRSA: Linezolid, vancomycin, daptomycin
  (Cubicin®)

(Cubicin®), linezolid (Zyvox®), tigecycline (Tygacil®), or vancomycin may need to be added or begun empirically, especially in institutions where MRSA is a frequent clinical isolate, in patients with positive MRSA cultures, or in patients at high risk for MRSA infection including those with previous MRSA infection, those who have been hospitalized or living in nursing homes, or those who have received multiple courses of different antibiotics over the previous 24 months. For less severe infections caused by MRSA, oral antibiotics such as trimethoprim/sulfamethoxazole (TMP/SMX) (Bactrim™, Septra®), doxycycline (Doryx®, Monodox®, Vibramycin®), or minocycline (Dynacin®, Minocin®) may be useful. Of these anti-MRSA antibiotics, only linezolid has been specifically studied in the diabetic foot infection and carries an FDA indication for the treatment of diabetic foot without concomitant osteomyelitis.

Milder soft-tissue infections of the diabetic foot may require no more than 10 to 14 days of antimicrobial therapy. More severe infections require longer therapy, especially if bone involvement is present. Limited ablative surgery to remove localized bone infection may decrease the duration of therapy and the incidence of relapse. If bone infection is not ablated completely, prolonged therapy (involving a minimum of 4 weeks of intravenous or 10 weeks of combined intravenous and oral therapy) may be required.

When dermatophyte infection is present (Figure 6-8, see color plate insert), topical antifungal agents should be used. In patients with more extensive fungal foot infection, oral therapy with itraconazole (Sporanox®) or fluconazole (Diflucan®) is effective. Toenail infection by a dermatophyte (onychomycosis) is more difficult to treat. Recurrences are common, and the decision to initiate therapy and which agent to use should be individualized. Options for therapy of onychomycosis include systemic antifungal agents (griseofulvin [Grifulvin V®], 750 to 1,000 mg daily for 4 to 6 months; terbinafine [Lamisil®], 250 mg daily for 12 weeks; or itraconazole [Sporanox®], pulse dosing 200 to 400 mg daily for 1 week each month, for 3 months), surgery, or chemical nail avulsion (40% urea preparation). Of the systemic antifungal agents, griseofulvin is no longer favored because of its associated side effects, including frequent headaches and GI disturbances, and the possibility of hepatotoxicity.

Other adjunctive therapies, such as hyperbaric oxygen (HBO) and tissue growth factors, have been shown to be effective, but large-scale, comparative clinical trials are not available.

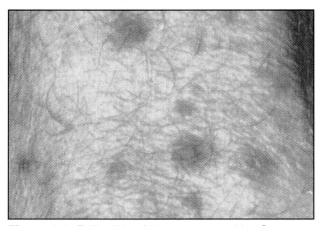

Figure 4-1: Folliculitis of the arm caused by *S aureus*.

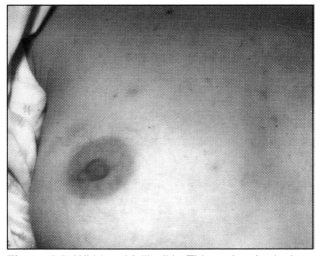

Figure 4-2: Whirlpool folliculitis. This patient had a low-grade fever associated with mastitis (erythema above the areola) and a generalized papular rash noted 2 days after using a hot tub at a resort hotel. The infection resolved within a few days.

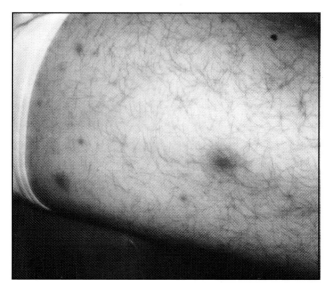

Figure 4-3: Furuncles and folliculitis caused by *S aureus* on the thigh of a dialysis patient.

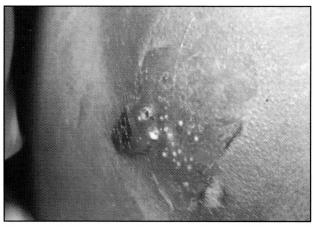

Figure 4-4: Carbuncle with surrounding cellulitis caused by *S aureus* on the back of a diabetic patient.

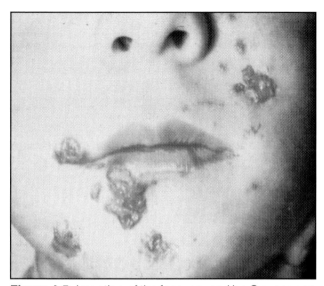

Figure 4-5: Impetigo of the face, caused by *S pyogenes*. The crusts, which are honey-colored, are typical. (Abner Kurtin, *Folica Dermatologica*, Geigy Pharmaceuticals)

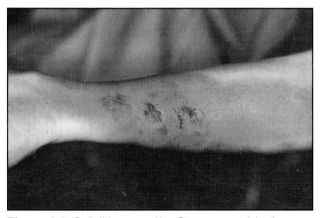

Figure 4-6: Cellulitis caused by *S pyogenes* of the forearm of a patient who had suffered abrasions in the area.

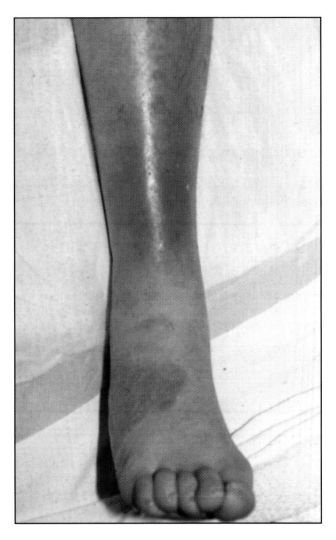

Figure 4-7: Cellulitis on the distal leg in a patient with recurrent psoriasis (note the area of psoriatic involvement on the dorsum of the foot).

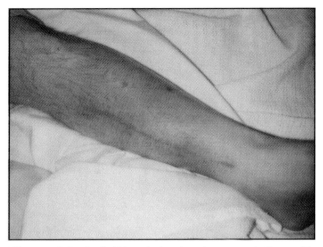

Figure 4-8: Cellulitis of the leg in association with vein donor site from prior coronary artery bypass graft (CABG) surgery. The patient also had tinea pedis.

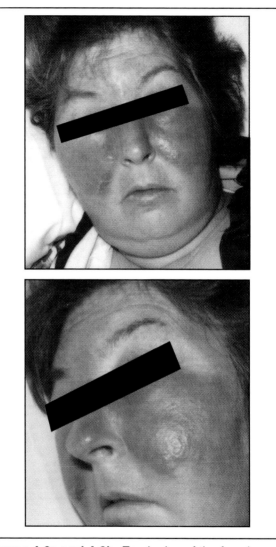

Figures 4-9a and 4-9b: Erysipelas of the face in a patient with positive blood cultures for *S pyogenes*.

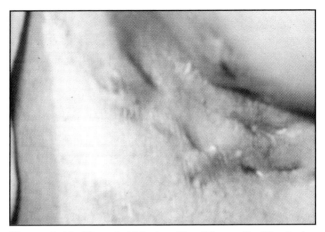

Figure 4-10: Chronic hidadrenitis of the axilla. The indurated areas and draining sinus tracts are typical.

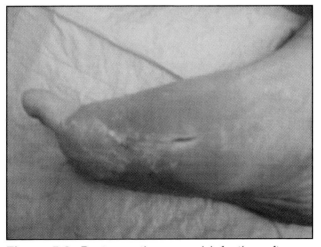

Figure 5-2: Postoperative wound infection after orthopedic surgery procedure; moderate erythema and induration are present.

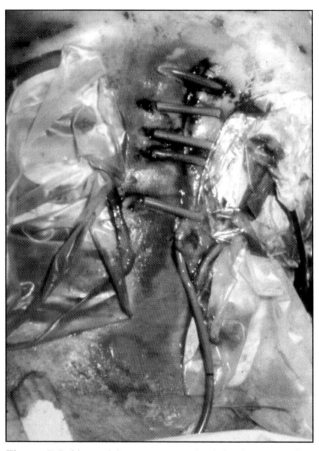

Figure 5-3: Necrotizing postoperative infection occurring after bowel surgery and associated with anastomic leak and polymicrobial infection.

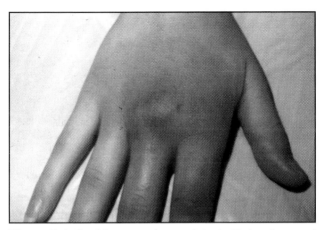

Figure 5-4: Cat bite wound associated with involvement of the metacarpophalangeal joint.

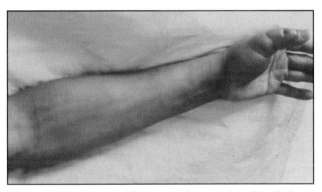

Figure 5-5: Human bite wound associated with lymphangitis.

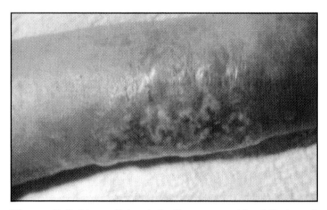

Figure 5-6: Necrotizing infection caused by *Vibrio vulnificus* in a patient who was cleaning crabs.

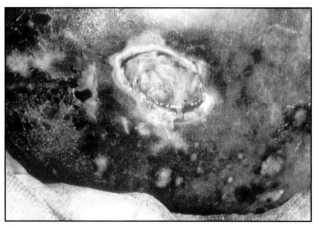

Figure 5-7: Infected decubitus ulcer.

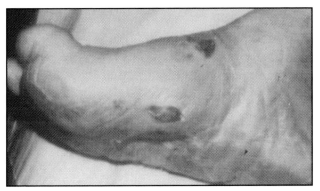

Figure 6-1: Diabetic neuropathy leading to loss of normal architecture (arch), resulting in 'flat foot.' This condition causes increased pressure on the skin overlying the metatarsal heads, often leading to ulcer formation.

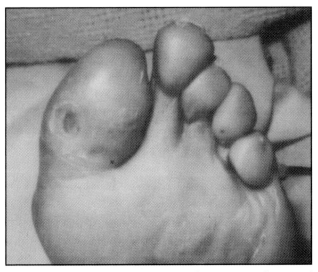

Figure 6-2: Superficial toe ulcer that occurred several days after the patient purchased new shoes, resulting in pressure blister and subsequent ulceration.

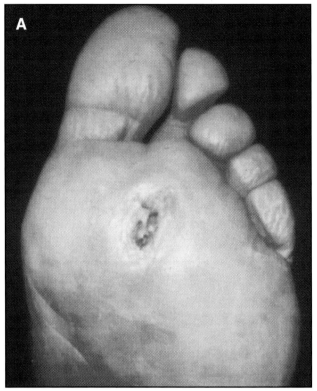

Figure 6-3a: Deep (central) space infection.

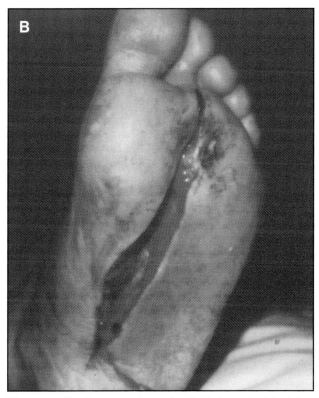

Figure 6-3b: Same patient after initial surgical incision and debridement.

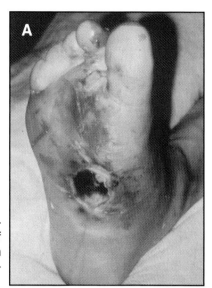

Figure 6-4a: Diabetic foot ulcer of 3 months' duration associated with osteomyelitis.

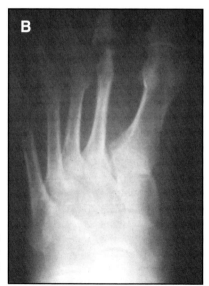

Figure 6-4b: Bone x-ray of same patient showing bone erosion.

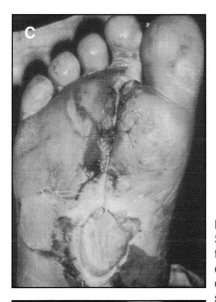

Figure 6-4c:
Same patient after excision of necrotic tissue and drainage of deep space.

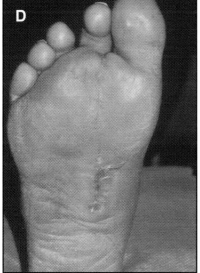

Figure 6-4d:
Same patient 6 weeks later.

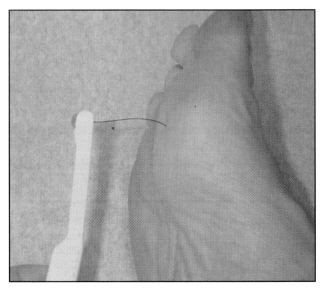

Figure 6-5: Monofilament used to test for sensation.

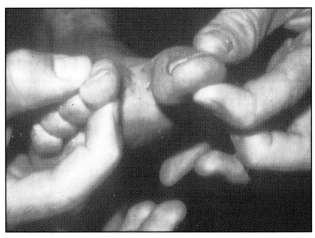

Figure 6-8: Tinea pedis is commonly found in diabetics and may precede bacterial infections.

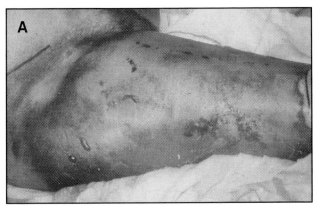

Figure 7-2a: Polymicrobial necrotizing fasciitis in a 60-year-old diabetic woman.

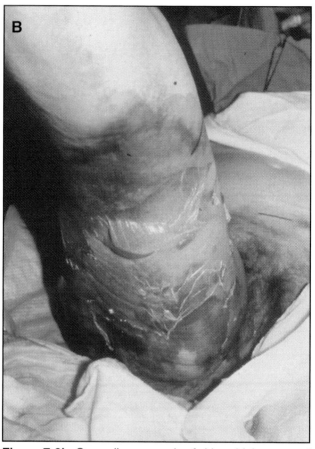

Figure 7-2b: Spreading necrosis of skin, which occurred over a 72-hour period.

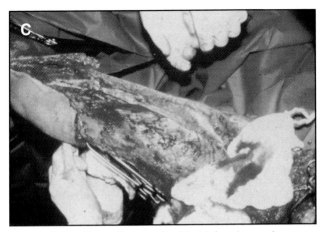

Figure 7-2c: Operative surgical field; fascia can be seen reflected over viable muscle.

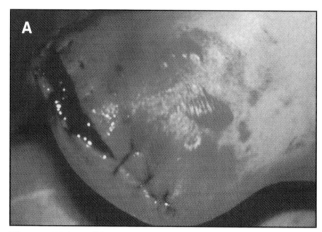

Figure 7-3a: *Clostridium* myonecrosis. Postoperative *Clostridium perfringens* gas gangrene occurring in a diabetic patient approximately 10 hours after elective lower extremity amputation.

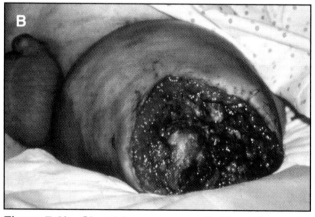

Figure 7-3b: *Clostridium* myonecrosis. Necrotic muscle in patient.

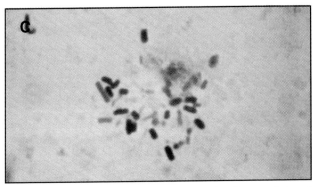

Figure 7-3c: *Clostridium* myonecrosis. Gram stain of drainage from the wound, showing large gram-positive (variable) bacilli and no polymorphonuclear leukocytes (PMNs).

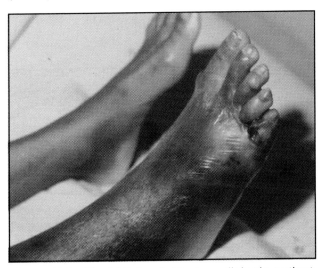

Figure 7-4: Clostridial cellulitis in a diabetic patient. There is abundance of gas, but the patient was not systemically ill. The patient was successfully treated with local debridement and penicillin.

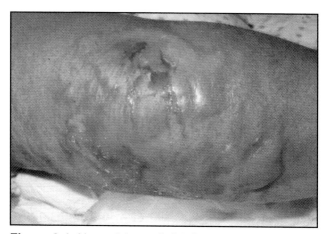

Figure 8-1: Necrotizing cellulitis/fasciitis of the elbow of a previously healthy 32-year-old woman who presented with *Streptococcus* toxic shock syndrome (TSS).

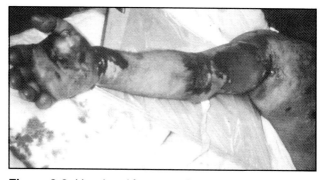

Figure 8-2: Hand and forearm of a 73-year-old man with group A *Streptococcus* (GAS) necrotizing fasciitis/myonecrosis. This patient was home eating dinner 6 hours before this photograph was taken, illustrating the rapid onset of severe and extensive disease. Amputation of the entire upper extremity was performed.

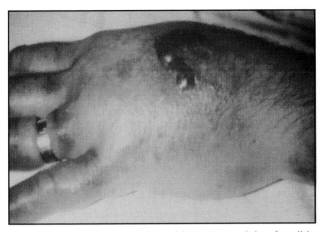

Figure 8-3: Bullous cellulitis without necrotizing fasciitis in a 60-year-old man.

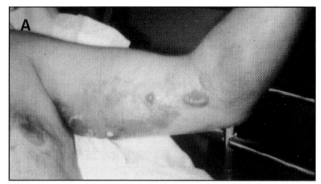

Figure 8-4a: Necrotizing fasciitis in a 67-year-old man.

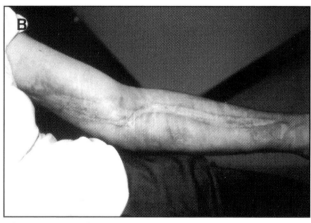

Figure 8-4b: Same patient after six operative procedures (fasciotomies and debridements).

Prevention

The prevention of infection is the cornerstone of diabetic foot care. The basic principles of such prevention include good control of the diabetic state, weight reduction, smoking avoidance, and a diet low in fat and cholesterol. Appropriate footwear is of paramount importance, and special shoes and/or orthotic devices may have to be made for diabetic patients, especially if they have foot deformities.

The most important factor in the prevention of lower extremity amputation is early detection of peripheral neuropathy. Patients who have lost the protection sensation in their feet are predisposed to repeated injuries and, therefore, to infection and amputation. Patients should be educated about the importance of glycemic control, proper foot care, and early reporting of foot problems. On the other hand, physicians should reinforce the importance of prevention by questioning patients about foot care and by performing a routine foot examination during each office visit. This examination should include checking for the presence or progression of neuropathy, pedal pulses, signs of microangiopathy, signs of irritation (ie, erythema), blister formation, calluses, ulcers, and foot architecture changes that may predispose the patient's feet to repeated pressure injury. The primary care physician should vigilantly look for any of these abnormal findings and then intervene promptly. A decision should be made to seek consultation with a foot and ankle specialist, a vascular surgeon, or a surgeon with special skills in the care of the diabetic foot if a patient's condition fails to respond to therapy. For hospitalized patients with foot infection, a team approach to care is appropriate. The primary care physician or the endocrinologist must be involved in monitoring metabolic needs and control of blood sugar. When the patient has a deep-tissue foot infection, consultation with an infectious disease specialist is strongly encouraged. In addition, these patients must be seen within 24 hours by a surgeon who is experienced in the care of diabetic foot problems.

6

Patients should take primary responsibility for their own foot care, inspecting their feet at least once daily. Hand mirrors may be used for this, and the help of family members or friends should be solicited if the patient's vision is too poor for adequate self-examination. The feet should be washed daily with nonmedicated soap and tepid water whose temperature was first tested with the fingers (but only if significant sensory neuropathy does not exist in the upper extremities as well). The feet, including the interdigital areas, should be dried thoroughly after washing, and then a light coat of lubricating lotion or talcum powder may be applied. Woolen socks should be used when the feet feel cold; hot water bottles or heating pads should never be used to warm the feet. To prevent ingrown toenails, the toenails should be cut straight across with nail clippers, without rounding at the corners. Ingrown toenails should be discussed with the patient's primary care physician and/or podiatrist.

Diabetic patients should avoid walking barefoot, either indoors or outdoors. They should also refrain from removing corns or calluses without professional help and from using caustic chemicals on their feet. Open-toed footwear should be avoided.

Primary care physicians should be familiar with their responsibilities to the diabetic patient. Physical examination for vascular and neurologic status should be performed at least twice yearly or more often if problems exist. Specialized examinations, such as Doppler studies, should be performed when indicated. Studies of shoe fitting and foot-loading patterns may be performed when necessary. Referral for a podiatric examination should be considered in all diabetic patients, especially those at higher risk for ulceration because of neuropathy, foot deformity, or a history of previous ulceration.

Summary

Foot infections in diabetics should be recognized and treated promptly. When superficial foot infections are treated before they spread, complications from costly deep-wound involvement can be avoided. Similarly, early recognition of deep-foot infections and timely surgical intervention of acute infection or infected foot ulcers are keys to good care. The physician should monitor risk factors that predispose a patient to infections, such as neuropathy, angiopathy, inadequate glycemic control, and poor foot hygiene.

We cannot emphasize enough the importance of prevention. Patient education is often lacking. Physicians neglect to do an adequate foot examination in the office and even in the hospital. The primary objectives in the management of diabetic foot infections are preservation and restoration of foot function. When a superficial infection is encountered, the physician should aggressively treat it to prevent progression to deeper tissues. When deep infection is suspected, surgical intervention and antibiotic treatment should be timely and aggressive. Prompt surgical debridement and even local amputation, together with antimicrobial therapy, will reduce limb loss and reduce the length of hospital stay. Many physicians who are not experienced in the care of these patients tend to take the approach of treating them medically with antibiotics alone and neglecting the benefit of surgical intervention. A team approach, including prompt surgical consultation for all patients hospitalized with foot infections, will provide better patient outcomes.

6

Selected Readings

Dang CN, Prasad YD, Boulton AJ, et al: Methicillin-resistant Staphylococcus aureus in the diabetic foot clinic: a worsening problem. *Diabet Med* 2003;20:159-161.

Eckman MH, Greenfield S, Mackey WC, et al: Foot infections in diabetic patients. Decision and cost-effectiveness analyses. *JAMA* 1995;273:712-720.

Frykberg RG, Armstrong DG, Giurini J, et al: Diabetic foot disorders: a clinical practice guideline. American College of Foot and Ankle Surgeons. *J Foot Ankle Surg* 2000;39(5 suppl):S1-S60.

Giordano P, Song J, Pertel P, et al: Sequential intravenous/oral moxifloxacin versus intravenous piperacillin-tazobactam followed by oral amoxicillin-clavulanate for the treatment of complicated skin and skin structure infection. *Int J Antimicrob Agents* 2005;26:357-365.

Grayson ML: Diabetic foot infections. Antimicrobial therapy. *Infect Dis Clin North Am* 1995;9:143-161.

Lavery LA, Armstrong DG, Vela SA, et al: Practical criteria for screening patients at high risk for diabetic foot ulceration. *Arch Intern Med* 1998;158:157-162.

Lipsky BA, Armstrong DG, Citron DM, et al: Ertapenem versus piperacillin/tazobactam for diabetic foot infections (SIDESTEP): prospective, randomised, controlled, double-blinded, multicentre trial. *Lancet* 2005;366:1695-1703.

Lipsky BA, Berendt AR, Deery HG, et al, and the Infectious Diseases Society of America: Diagnosis and treatment of diabetic foot infections. *Clin Infect Dis* 2004;39:885-910.

Lipsky BA, Itani K, Norden C: Treating foot infections in diabetic patients: a randomized, multicenter, open-label trial of linezolid versus ampicillin-sulbactam/amoxicillin-clavulanate. *Clin Infect Dis* 2004;38:17-24.

Lipsky BA: Osteomyelitis of the foot in diabetic patients. *Clin Infect Dis* 1997;25:1318-1326.

Tan JS, Anderson JL, Watanakunakorn C, et al: Neutrophil dysfunction in diabetes mellitus. *J Lab Clin Med* 1975;85:26-33.

Tan JS, File TM Jr: Diagnosis and treatment of diabetic foot infections. *Baillieres Best Pract Res Clin Rheumatol* 1999;13:149-161.

Tan JS, Friedman NM, Hazelton-Miller C, et al: Can aggressive treatment of diabetic foot infections reduce the need for above-ankle amputation? *Clin Infect Dis* 1996;23:286-291.

Chapter 7

Necrotizing Soft-Tissue Infections

N ecrotizing soft-tissue infections include skin and skin-structure infections characterized by necrosis of the skin, subcutaneous tissue, and fascia or muscle. These infections occur less frequently than pyodermas but require an aggressive early response for optimal management. They often progress quickly and dramatically, and frequently require urgent, aggressive surgical excision of tissue. Necrotizing infections are often deep and devastating, can cause major destruction of tissue, and may lead to death.

Necrotizing cutaneous infections are generally classified by selected characteristics such as necrotizing fasciitis, *Clostridium* myonecrosis, and synergistic necrotizing cellulitis (Table 7-1). However, initial clinical manifestations may not be distinct. We agree with others that classification into precise categories is often difficult and not relevant to the initial management of the patient.

Etiology

Necrotizing soft-tissue infections can be classified by etiology as either polymicrobial (involving mixed aerobes and anaerobes) or monomicrobial.

Polymicrobial Necrotizing Soft-tissue Infections

Polymicrobial infections are commonly found in the perineal area and lower extremities. In such cases, the fecal flora contribute to other skin pathogens. Gram-positive organisms,

Table 7-1: Characteristics of Severe Necrotizing Soft-Tissue Infections

	Anaerobic Gas-Forming Cellulitis	Synergistic Necrotizing Cellulitis
Predisposing condition	Trauma	Diabetes, prior local lesions, perirectal lesions
Incubation	>3 days	3 to 14 days
Etiology	Clostridia, others	Mixed aerobes, anaerobes
Systemic toxicity	Minimal	Moderate to severe
Course	Gradual	Acute
Local pain	Minimal	Moderate to severe
Skin appearance	Swollen, minimal discoloration	Erythematous or gangrenous
Gas	Abundant	Variable
Muscle involvement	No	Variable
Discharge	Thin, dark, sweetish or foul odor	Dark pus or 'dishwater,' putrid
Gram stain	PMNs, gram-positive bacilli	PMNs, mixed flora
Surgical therapy	Debridement	Wide-filleting incisions

PMNs=polymorphonuclear leukocytes
Modified from Gorbach, 1996.

Gas Gangrene	**Streptococcal Myonecrosis**
Trauma or surgical wound	Trauma, surgery
1 to 4 days	3 to 4 days
Clostridia, especially *C perfringens*	Anaerobic streptococci
Severe	Minimal until late in course
Acute	Subacute
Severe	Late only
Tense and blanched yellow-bronze, necrotic with hemorrhagic bullae	Erythematous or yellow-bronze
Usually present	Variable
Myonecrosis	Myonecrosis
Serosanguineous, sweet or foul odor	Seropurulent
Sparse PMNs, gram-positive bacilli	PMNs, gram-positive bacilli
Extensive excision, amputation	Excision of necrotic muscle

7

(continued on next page)

Table 7-1: Characteristics of Severe Necrotizing Soft-Tissue Infections *(continued)*

	Necrotizing Fasciitis	Infected Vascular Gangrene
Predisposing condition	Diabetes, trauma, surgery, perineal infection	Arterial insufficiency
Incubation	1 to 4 days	>5 days
Etiology	Type I: polymicrobial (aerobic/anaerobic) Type II: *S pyogenes*	Mixed aerobes, anaerobes
Systemic toxicity	Moderate to severe	Minimal
Course	Acute to subacute	Subacute
Local pain	Minimal to moderate	Variable
Skin appearance	Blanched, erythematous, necrotic with hemorrhagic bullae	Erythematous or necrotic
Gas	Variable	Variable
Muscle involvement	No	Myonecrosis limited to area of vascular insufficiency
Discharge	Seropurulent 'dishwater,' putrid	Minimal
Gram stain	Gram-positive cocci	PMNs, mixed flora
Surgical therapy	Wide-filleting incisions	Amputation

PMNs=polymorphonuclear leukocytes
Modified from Gorbach, 1996.

such as *Staphylococcus* species, *Streptococcus* species, or *Enterococcus* species, gram-negative enteric bacilli, and anaerobes are frequently isolated from such infections. In combination, these bacteria may induce the formation of abscesses as well as severe necrotizing infections.

The pathogenic role of mixed aerobic/anaerobic infections has been well demonstrated in a number of animal models of infection (Figures 7-1a and 7-1b). In 1974, Weinstein et al first published results of a peritonitis/intra-abdominal abscess model in rats that demonstrated a biphasic infection. The first phase was manifested by peritonitis caused by facultative aerobes, while in the second phase, anaerobes were predominant. In an animal model that more closely mimics skin and soft-tissue infection, Brook evaluated the effect of inoculating various combinations or aerobes and anaerobes subcutaneously into mice. Mice were challenged with either a single organism or a mixture of *Bacteroides* species and facultative aerobic organisms. The bacterial strains tested included *Bacteroides fragilis, Escherichia coli, Bacteroides melaninogenicus, Klebsiella pneumoniae, Pseudomonas aeruginosa, Staphylococcus aureus, Streptococcus pyogenes,* and *Enterococcus faecalis* (all of which are commonly found in mixed aerobic/anaerobic skin and soft-tissue infections in humans). Infection caused by individual isolates was relatively innocuous, but combinations of facultative organisms and aerobes showed a synergistic effect, as manifested by the formation of abscesses and by significant increased animal mortality. This synergistic effect was demonstrated between the *Bacteroides* species and all of the tested facultative aerobic organisms. The effect was also seen between most peptostreptococci, *P aeruginosa*, and *S aureus*.

Brook electively treated inoculated animals with a variety of antibiotics chosen to cover specific aerobes, anaerobes, or both. Antimicrobial agents aimed at one component of a mixed infection did not eliminate the infection or eradicate the untreated organisms, so abscesses persisted.

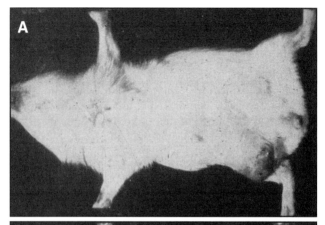

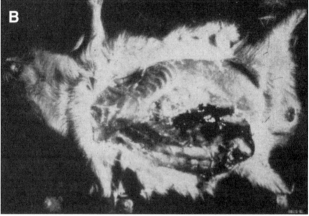

Figure 7-1: Animal model of synergistic infection.
A: Intracutaneous inoculation of single organism caused mild infection.
B: Inoculation of combination of organisms produced a more virulent, necrotizing, spreading infection. From MacDonald JB, Sutton RM, Knoll ML: The production of fusospirochetal infections in guinea pigs with recombined pure cultures. *J Infect Dis* 1954;95:275-284. Used with permission.

Therapy aimed at both components was required to achieve a significant reduction in the number of both contributing pathogens. Using another soft-tissue infection model, Kelly demonstrated synergy between *E coli* and *B fragilis* when injected subcutaneously into guinea pigs. A certain threshold of numbers of organisms was required for this synergistic effect to occur. When the number of *E coli* or *B fragilis* inocula was less than a critical threshold (10^4 *B fragilis* or 10^3 *E coli*), no abscess with necrosis occurred; above the threshold number, significant bacterial growth, abscess formation, and necrosis were observed.

These animal studies and others tend to confirm the observation that mixed aerobic/anaerobic infections are often more virulent than monomicrobial infections caused by the same organisms. Mackowiak has identified several factors that allow micro-organisms to interact and produce a synergistic infection:

- An effect on host defenses (most commonly inhibition of phagocytosis)
- Supplementation of vital nutrients
- Provision of environmental conditions favorable for growth
- Increased virulence of the organisms

Monomicrobial Necrotizing Soft-tissue Infections

Several individual pathogens may cause necrotizing soft-tissue infections. Most significant are those caused by *Clostridium* species and *S pyogenes*.

Clostridia may play a role in various infections of skin, subcutaneous tissue, and muscle, including crepitant cellulitis, pyomyositis, and clostridial myonecrosis (gas gangrene). *Clostridium perfringens* is the major causative species and accounts for approximately 80% of cases. Other *Clostridium* species include *Clostridium septicum*, *Clostridium novyi*, *Clostridium sordellii*, *Clostridium histolyticum*, and *Clostridium bifermentans*. Implicated *Clostridium* species produce various exotoxins that contribute to the pathophysiology of necrotizing soft-tissue infections. *Clostridium* are anaerobic, and, therefore, require an anaerobic environment for multiplication and production of their necrotizing toxins. Clostridia can be either endogenous or exogenous in origin because they may be present in a patient's normal gastrointestinal (GI) flora or may occur from soil contamination, such as in wounds that result from trauma (ie, motorcycle or lawn mower accidents).

Over the past decade, there have been increasing reports of necrotizing fasciitis caused by group A *Streptococcus* (GAS) and *S pyogenes*. In addition to GAS and *Clostridium* species, other pathogens that may cause necrotizing fasciitis include *Staphylococcus* species (ie, community-acquired *Staphyloccus aureus* [CA-MRSA]), *Vibrio vulnificus* (salt water injury), *Aeromonas hydrophila* (fresh water injury), Enterobacteriaceae, *P aeruginosa*, and *Yersinia enterocolitica*.

Clinical Manifestations

Clinical features that suggest necrotizing soft-tissue infections include:

- Severe, constant pain
- Bullous lesions
- Gas in soft tissues that is detected by palpation, radiographs, or scanning. The gases are produced by metabolic activity of the aerobic and/or anaerobic bacteria. When anaerobes are present, there is often a distinctive putrid odor.
- Systemic toxicity manifested by fever and, occasionally, delirium
- Tendency for rapid spread centrally along the fascial planes

Inflammatory reaction to such infections is often much different from that seen in the pyodermas caused by staphylococci; rather than purulent discharge associated with abscess formation, there is often a serous, putrid, dishwaterlike discharge.

Necrotizing soft-tissue infections frequently occur in association with previous trauma, surgery, or other forms of tissue damage. Diabetes is a common underlying condition. Infections associated with pre-existing ulcers (ie, diabetic foot ulcers or decubitus ulcers) may progress to necrotizing infections. Tissue necrosis is characteristic and can occur by any one of several means: pressure necrosis from infected areas contained by fascia or skin; vascular thrombosis produced by anaerobic organisms secondary to heparinized production or by direct acceleration of coagulation; and extracellular toxins produced by bacteria, such as the necrotoxins of *C perfringens*. The clinical characteristics of the more common necrotizing soft-tissue infections are listed in Table 7-1. Many of these conditions are differentiated based on the anatomical extent of disease, which is often determined only at the time of surgical intervention. A look at additional salient clinical features of necrotizing soft-tissue infections follows.

Polymicrobial Infections

Necrotizing fasciitis refers to deep-tissue infection involving the fascial cleft between the subcutaneous tissue and underlying muscle. Necrotizing fasciitis is an uncommon soft-tissue infection characterized by rapidly spreading inflammation and subsequent necrosis of the muscle fascia and overlying skin. This potentially life-threatening infection is usually grouped under the larger classification of necrotizing soft-tissue infections, which are differentiated by the anatomic extent of involvement, and include clostridial cellulitis, synergistic necrotizing cellulitis, and gas gangrene (myonecrosis). Necrotizing fasciitis usually involves extensive inflammation of subcutaneous tissue that progressively destroys fascia and fat, but spares the muscle (Figures 7-2a to 7-2c, see color plate insert). Extension to the muscle (ie, streptococcal myositis or myonecrosis) may occur with necrotizing fasciitis, but is less common. Previous descriptions of necrotizing fasciitis have classified patients as one of two types: type I are patients with polymicrobial, mixed anaerobic/aerobic microbiology; type II are patients with *S pyogenes* as the predominant pathogen. Until recently, most reviews of necrotizing fasciitis have focused on patients with anaerobic/polymicrobial infection (type I) often in association with underlying conditions such as diabetes. Overlying cutaneous necrosis often occurs secondary to the ischemic effects of vascular thrombosis. The most distinguishing clinical feature is the wooden, hard feel of the subcutaneous tissues. In cellulitis or erysipelas, the subcutaneous tissues yield under palpation. But in fasciitis, the underlying tissues are firm and the fascial planes and muscle groups cannot be discerned by palpation. It is often possible to observe a broader erythematous track of the skin along the route of the fascial plane as the infection advances. If there is an open wound, probing the edges with a blunt instrument permits ready dissection of the superficial fascial planes well beyond the wound margins. Remarkably little pain may be associated with this procedure because of anesthesia that occurs secondary to necrosis of nerve endings. Infection of the fascial cleft may spread rapidly; however, on occasion, it may be indolent.

Fournier's gangrene is a form of necrotizing fasciitis that involves the fascial planes of the scrotum perineum. It may spread to the abdominal wall or thighs.

Synergistic necrotizing cellulitis is similar to type I necrotizing fasciitis in that both are caused by a mixed aerobic/anaerobic infection; however, with necrotizing cellulitis, there is often extension beneath the fascia involving muscle. Just as in clostridial myonecrosis, amputation is required when there is muscle involvement of an extremity.

Progressive bacterial synergistic gangrene (often referred to as Meleney's gangrene) is an indolent process characterized by poor healing, often after a previous surgical operation. The presentation may be a slowly progressive (often over several weeks) expanding necrosis. Local pain and tenderness are nearly always present, but fever and systemic toxicity are not, as they are with the other syndromes.

Pyomyositis is a discrete abscess within individual muscle groups caused primarily by *S aureus* but occasionally by other gram-positive organisms or gram-negative enteric rods. Because of its geographic distribution, this condition is often referred to as tropical pyomyositis, but cases are increasingly recognized in temperate climates, especially in patients with human immunodeficiency virus (HIV) or diabetes. The presenting signs are localized pain in a single muscular group, muscle spasm, and fever. The disease most often occurs in an extremity, but any muscle group may be involved. Additionally, it may not be possible to palpate a discrete abscess because the infection is localized deep within the muscle, but the area has a firm, woody feel upon palpation, along with pain and tenderness.

Clostridial Necrotizing Infections

The clinical picture of clostridial myonecrosis, or classic gas gangrene, is well described. Clostridial myonecrosis may occur within hours of an initiating insult or surgery, and is often associated with sudden pain that increases in severity and extends beyond the wound. Systemic toxicity indicated by tachycardia and mental confusion is common. A thin, watery discharge is often noted early in the process; large hemorrhagic bullae may appear in the vicinity of the wound (Figures 7-3a and 7-3b, see color plate insert). Microscopic examination of the discharge often reveals gram-positive rods and a paucity of polymorphonuclear leukocytes (PMNs) (Figure 7-3c, see color plate insert). The lack of PMNs is, in part, attributable to clostridial toxins that lyse white blood cell membranes and cause subsequent cell death. The characteristic finding of clostridial myonecrosis is the appearance of necrotic, infected muscle. As the disease progresses, the muscle loses viability and becomes black. Early diagnosis is essential so that complete resection (amputation) of the devitalized tissue can be accomplished.

Although classic gangrene implies infection by *Clostridium* species, the isolation of *Clostridium* species (eg, *C perfringens*) does not necessarily indicate clinical disease. This is because *Clostridium* species (including *C perfringens*) commonly colonize or contaminate wounds (either postsurgical or post-traumatic) without causing tissue invasion. In addition, *C perfringens* may cause only cellulitis (anaerobic cellulitis) without deep-tissue involvement. In such cases, there may be an abundance of gas formation but severe pain and systemic toxicity are absent (Figure 7-4, see color plate insert).

Diagnosis

Although the diagnosis of necrotizing fasciitis and other necrotizing soft-tissue infections may be clear-cut at the later stage of disease (extensive necrosis), it is often difficult to differentiate from primary cellulitis early in presentation. The distinction is important because cellulitis can be treated with antimicrobial agents without surgical management, while deep necrotizing soft-tissue infections require timely surgical debridement and excision of tissue in addition to the use of antimicrobial agents.

Clinical characteristics that should direct physicians to consider deep necrotizing soft-tissue infections are listed in Table 7-2. Bullae may be observed in cellulitis without fasciitis. Bullae may also be associated with toxins (eg, brown recluse spider bites), and primarily dermatologic conditions (eg, pyoderma gangrenosum). However, fever with unexplained severe musculoskeletal pain is an important clue to imminent necrotizing fasciitis. Other conditions that may mimic the early manifestations of necrotizing soft-tissue infections include trauma with hematoma (although fever and leukocytosis are usually absent), phlebitis, bursitis, and arthritis. In addition, noninfectious processes can be associated with the presence of gas in subcutaneous tissue: (1) subcutaneous emphysema secondary to local

Table 7-2: Characteristics of Necrotizing Soft-Tissue Infection (When to Suspect Necrotizing Fasciitis or Other Necrotizing Infection Rather Than Cellulitis)

- Severe pain
- Rapidly spreading swelling and inflammation
- Pain followed by anesthesia
- Bullous formation
- Necrosis (later appearance)
- Toxic shock syndrome (TSS)
- Laboratory-elevated creatinine phosphokinase (CPK)
- Adequate debridement can rarely be performed in one step

trauma or after surgical procedures, (2) use of H_2O_2, and (3) introduction of air during irrigation.

Leukocytosis is usually present in most deep necrotizing soft-tissue infections. Gram-stain smears from aspirates or debrided tissue often reveal causative organisms (ie, gram-positive cocci for group A necrotizing fasciitis). In contrast, in our experience, a Gram stain is rarely positive in most cases of non-necrotizing cellulitis. An elevated serum creatinine phosphokinase (CPK) level is often a clue to the presence of necrotizing fasciitis or myositis. Blood cultures are frequently positive in necrotizing soft-tissue infections. Kaul et al found that bacteremia predicted increased mortality in necrotizing fasciitis; however, bacteremia is not a clinically useful marker because it can be detected only 24 to 48 hours after presentation. Similarly, the presence of GAS bacteremia does not reliably distinguish necrotizing fasciitis from cellulitis because bacteremia is also found in association with non-necrotizing cellulitis.

7

The most definitive diagnostic test is therapeutic surgical exploration to define the extent of infection in the involved tissues (ie, subcutaneous, fascia, muscle). Whenever necrotizing skin infection is considered in the differential diagnosis, an immediate surgical evaluation is imperative. Diagnostic studies before surgical incision and drainage may include radiography, which may demonstrate soft-tissue swelling or the presence of gas; computed tomography (CT) scan or ultrasound to detect fluid or abscesses, for which needle aspiration may be directed; and biopsy. CT, magnetic resonance imaging (MRI), and routine soft-tissue roentgenogram may help in demonstrating the involvement of subcutaneous tissue beyond the visibly involved cutaneous abnormality. GAS in tissue favors mixed aerobic/anaerobic infection or gas gangrene caused by clostridia. GAS do not produce gas. However, these studies should not delay surgical evaluation if necrotizing soft-tissue infection is suspected. Rather, they should serve to expedite and direct surgical intervention.

Treatment

The approach to management of necrotizing soft-tissue infections requires expeditious evaluation, with early surgical intervention. The mortality rate of necrotizing fasciitis approaches 100% if appropriate surgical intervention is not performed, and it correlates with timing of surgery. Thus, regardless of the microbial etiology, the primary therapy is urgent surgery accompanied with antibiotics active against the most likely pathogens (ie, streptococci, staphylococci, enterococci, *Clostridium* species, and mixed aerobic/anaerobic flora) (Table 7-3).

Surgery

The goals of surgery are threefold: (1) to remove all necrotic tissue by radical debridement, (2) to preserve as much viable skin as possible, and (3) to maintain hemostasis. Amputation may be necessary to remove all nonviable

Table 7-3: Recommended Initial Therapy for Necrotizing Soft-Tissue Infections

- Surgical debridement/amputation
- Antimicrobial therapy: piperacillin/tazobactam (Zosyn®IV), ticarcillin/clavulanate (Timentin®), or imipenem/cilastatin (Primaxin®) *plus* clindamycin (see text for explanation)
- For penicillin-allergic patients: clindamycin (Cleocin®) *plus* ciprofloxacin (Cipro®, ProQuin® XR) or levofloxacin (Levaquin®)
- Tetanus toxoid
  - for severe cases: intravenous immunoglobulin (IVIG)
- Value of hyperbaric oxygen is controversial

tissues (this is particularly important for myonecrosis). A second-look procedure may be (and often is) necessary within 12 to 24 hours to reculture and remove all necrotic and infected materials that may have been missed. Multiple debridements may be necessary. General principles in the care of necrotizing fasciitis, which apply to many other necrotizing soft-tissue infections, are listed in Table 7-4.

Empiric Antimicrobial Therapy

It is difficult to determine the microbial etiology on the basis of clinical presentation; therefore, empiric antibiotic therapy should be started as soon as this disease is suspected. The antimicrobial agents chosen should have activity against streptococci, staphylococci, *Clostridium*, and mixed aerobic/anaerobic organisms. The combination of a β-lactam/β-lactamase inhibitor, such as ticarcillin/clavulanate (Timentin®) or piperacillin/tazobactam (Zosyn®IV), or a carbapenem (imipenem/cilastatin [Primaxin®] or meropenem [Merrem®, Merrem®IV]), should provide adequate spectrum.

Table 7-4: General Principles in the Care of Patients With Necrotizing Fasciitis

- Patients with necrotizing fasciitis or myonecrosis who do not undergo exploration and debridement will surely die.
- Devitalized tissue, including muscle, fascia, and skin, must be removed.
- Appropriate surgical debridement in certain locations of the body—head, neck, thorax, abdomen—may be virtually impossible.
- Multiple debridements over the course of several weeks are usually necessary.
- Extensive reconstructive surgery is generally necessary.

Some Corollaries to These Principles

- Adequate debridement can rarely be performed in one step.
- Skin overlying necrotic fascia may remain viable, and if it appears to be so at the time of initial debridement, it may be spared for a second look during follow-up debridement.
- Patients with established necrotizing fasciitis are frequently poor surgical risks, with high surgical mortality and morbidity; nonetheless, failure to perform the operation will result in virtually 100% mortality.
- If primary care physicians are concerned that a deeper infection might be present, surgical evaluation is warranted.

Adapted from Stevens DL: Necrotizing fasciitis: do not wait to make a diagnosis. *Infect Med* 1997;14:684-688.

Because of the presence of a large inoculum of bacteria (such that a high percentage of organisms may not be in a logarithmic phase of growth), penicillin and other β-lactam antibiotics may not be very effective. Further, Stevens et al demonstrated that streptococci do not express penicillin-binding proteins (PBPs) on their membranes during the stationary phase, that is, when they are not dividing. Clindamycin (Cleocin®), in contrast, has shown greater efficacy in experimental formidable streptococcal infection. Clindamycin, unlike the β-lactams, inhibits protein synthesis and is not affected by the inoculum size or the stage of bacterial growth. In addition, clindamycin suppresses bacterial toxin synthesis and enhances phagocytosis of streptococci.

We recommend initial therapy with a combination of a β-lactam/β-lactamase inhibitor and clindamycin until the etiology is known. For penicillin-allergic patients, a combination of clindamycin and a fluoroquinolone can be used. Tetanus prophylaxis should be administered in patients who are not up to date with immunizations (Table 7-3).

Historically, *S aureus* has not caused necrotizing fasciitis; however, recent community-acquired methicillin-resistant *S aureus* (CA-MRSA) strains that contain the gene for Panton-Valentine leukocidin (PVL) cytotoxin have caused necrotizing fasciitis.

Other Therapies

HBO is controversial as a therapy for necrotizing soft-tissue infections. HBO has long been recommended for the treatment of clostridial myonecrosis and more recently has been applied to other necrotizing infections. However, the role of HBO is, at best, adjunctive. The benefits are far clearer in *Clostridium* myonecrosis than in other necrotizing infections because HBO is bactericidal for *C perfringens* and may reduce the generation of exotoxin in *Clostridium* myonecrosis (but it will not neutralize toxin already present). Experimental studies have not demonstrated the efficacy of HBO. HBO should be limited to specialized centers where complications can be kept to a minimum, and it should never take precedence over surgical debridement.

IVIG has been shown to have some beneficial effect in toxic shock syndrome (TSS) associated with GAS necrotizing fasciitis (see Chapter 8). This effect may be due to its ability to neutralize superantigen.

Prevention

Because necrotizing soft-tissue infections often occur as complications of less serious cutaneous infections (ie, diabetic lower extremity ulcers), clinicians should focus their attention on preventing pressure ulcers and wounds in patients with identifiable risk factors. Patients with conditions such as diabetes must be educated about their predisposition to infections and alerted to the early signs of infection. Early treatment of superficial infections in such patients can ward off the serious complication of necrotizing, deep soft-tissue infections.

Selected Readings

Bodemer C, Panhans A, Chretien-Marquet B, et al: Staphylococcal necrotizing fasciitis in the mammary region in childhood: a report of five cases. *J Pediatr* 1997;131:466-469.

Brook I: Synergistic aerobic and anaerobic infections. *Clin Ther* 1987; 20(suppl A):19-35.

File TM Jr, Tan JS: The triple threat of gram-positive cocci, gram-negative bacilli, and anaerobes. In: Nord CE, ed: *The Role of Piperacillin/Tazobactam in the Treatment of Skin and Soft-Tissue Infections*. Montreal, Canada, PharmaLibri, 1994.

File TM, Jr, Tan JS: Treatment of necrotizing soft tissue infections. *Compl Surg* 1993;(suppl):43-49.

Furusu A, Yoshizuka N, Abe K, et al: *Aeromonas hydrophila* necrotizing fasciitis and gas gangrene in a diabetic patient on haemodialysis. *Nephrol Dial Transplant* 1997;12:1730-1734.

Gardam M, Low DE, Saginur R, et al: Group B streptococcal necrotizing fasciitis and streptococcal toxic shock-like syndrome in adults. *Arch Intern Med* 1998;158:1704-1708.

Giuliano A, Lewis F, Hadley K, et al: Bacteriology of necrotizing fasciitis. *Am J Surg* 1977;134:52-57.

Gorbach SL: IDCP Guidelines: necrotizing skin and soft tissue infections. Part I: necrotizing fasciitis. *Infect Dis Clin Pract* 1996;5:406-411.

Gorbach SL: IDCP Guidelines: necrotizing skin and soft tissue infections. Part II: myositis, Meleney's gangrene, pyomyositis, necrotizing cellulitis, nonclostridial cellulitis, and Fournier's gangrene. *Infect Dis Clin Pract* 1996;5:463-472.

Halow KD, Harner RC, Fontenelle LJ: Primary skin infections secondary to *Vibrio vulnificus*: the role of operative intervention. *J Am Coll Surg* 1996;183:329-334.

Kelly MJ: The quantitative and histological demonstration of pathogenic synergy between *Escherichia coli* and *Bacteroides fragilis* in guinea pig wounds. *J Med Microbiol* 1978;11:513-523.

Lewis RT: Necrotizing soft-tissue infections. *Infect Dis Clin North Am* 1992;6:693-703.

MacDonald JB, Sutton RM, Knoll ML: The production of fusospirochetal infections in guinea pigs with recombined pure cultures. *J Infect Dis* 1954;95:275-284.

Mackowiak PA: Microbial synergism in human infections (second of two parts). *N Engl J Med* 1978;298:83-87.

Schreuder F, Chatoo M: Another cause of necrotizing fasciitis? *J Infect* 1997;35:177-178.

Stevens DL: Necrotizing fasciitis: don't wait to make a diagnosis. *Infect Med* 1997;14:684-688.

Stevens DL, Gibbons AE, Bergstrom R, et al: The Eagle effect revisited: efficacy of clindamycin, erythromycin, and penicillin in the treatment of streptococcal myositis. *J Infect Dis* 1988;158:23-28.

Stevens DL, Yan S, Bryant AE: Penicillin-binding protein expression at different growth stages determines penicillin efficacy in vitro and in vivo: an explanation for the inoculum effect. *J Infect Dis* 1993;167:1401-1405.

Swartz MN: Cellulitis and subcutaneous tissue infections. In: Mandell GL, Bennett JE, Dolin R, eds: *Principles and Practice of Infectious Diseases*, 4th ed. Philadelphia, WB Saunders, 1995, pp 909-929.

Weinstein WM, Onderdonk AB, Bartlett JG, et al: Experimental intra-abdominal abscesses in rats: development of an experimental model. *Infect Immunol* 1974;10:1250-1255.

7

Chapter 8

Group A *Streptococcus* Necrotizing Fasciitis

T he incidence of invasive group A *Streptococcus* (GAS) infections (including necrotizing fasciitis) has increased in the past decade, raising awareness of this dangerous pathogen. Because GAS necrotizing fasciitis has the potential to rapidly destroy tissue, the lay press has dramatically designated this disease as the flesh-eating bacteria syndrome.

Recent Perspectives of GAS Necrotizing Fasciitis

Streptococcus pyogenes is ubiquitous and is found in humans and animals. It is one of the most common human pathogens. In addition to pharyngitis and pyodermas, *S pyogenes* is associated with numerous infections, including scarlet fever, cellulitis, toxic shock syndrome (TSS), and necrotizing soft-tissue infections, as well as postinfectious sequelae such as rheumatic fever and acute glomerulonephritis. Fluctuations in the incidence and severity of these infections, particularly scarlet fever, have been common in the past. However, a dramatic decline in serious GAS infections occurred in the early 20th century and continued unabated until the mid-1980s, when invasive GAS infection re-emerged.

Pathophysiology: Virulence Factors

The recent increase in the number of reported invasive GAS infections re-emphasizes the pathogenic potential of this organism. Investigators have increased their efforts to uncover the virulence factors, both old and new, which may be responsible for the resurgence of severe disease. A number of GAS products, such as surface components and extracellular products, are believed to play important roles, including M-proteins, hyaluronic acid capsules, pyrogenic exotoxins, and additional excreted proteins that are produced by many, if not all, strains of GAS. Stevens et al recently discovered a strong association between isolates from invasive GAS infections and the production of NADase.

M-protein is believed to contribute to the invasiveness of the organism by its ability to resist phagocytosis. The production of type-specific antibody directed against a specific M-protein following infection is known to confer host resistance to GAS of that M-type. A major shift in the distribution of M-protein types was observed in the early 1980s, with an increasing frequency of M_1 and M_3 serotypes. Although these types were more often found in invasive fatal infections than other M-serotypes, other M-serotypes have also been recovered, including M_6, M_{12}, M_{18}, and M_{28}, as well as many nontypeable M-protein strains.

Initial studies of M_1 and M_3 isolates from invasive cases implicated streptococcal pyrogenic exotoxins (SPE), formerly known as erythrogenic or scarlet fever toxins. SPE A appears to play a major role in severe disease. A higher percentage of streptococcal isolates from invasive disease cases were shown to produce SPE A than strains from less severe disease cases.

Streptococcal pyrogenic exotoxins (ie, SPE A, SPE B, SPE C) belong to a group of proteins called superantigens. Superantigens are generally able to activate a much larger proportion of T cells than conventional peptide antigens in some patients, resulting in the production of various cytokines. These cytokines, in turn, are believed to be responsible for the manifestations of streptococcal TSS and necrotizing fasciitis. SPE A and SPE B induce mononuclear cells to produce cytokines (eg, tumor necrosis factor-α

8

[TNF-α], interleukin-1β [IL-β], interleukin-6 [IL-6]), which can mediate the fever, shock, and tissue injury observed with streptococcal TSS and necrotizing fasciitis. There is good evidence that cytokines play an important role in streptococcal TSS and necrotizing fasciitis. TNF-α, IL-1β, and IL-6 have been detected in the blood of patients with these conditions. Similarly, the administration of an anti-TNF-α monoclonal antibody improved survival in an animal model of TSS. Two newly described exotoxins, streptococcal superantigen (SSA) and mitogenic factor (MF), are also both capable of inducing a variety of cytokines.

The complex interaction between streptococcal virulence factors and the immune or nonimmune host ultimately determines the clinical syndrome and outcome of streptococcal infection. The quantity of virulence factors produced also contributes to the severity of illness. Recent evidence suggests that clonal expansion of more virulent strains of GAS may not be responsible for the increase in severe cases. Acquired immunity to one or more streptococcal virulence factors by most of the population has probably prevented large outbreaks of invasive disease. From 1994 to 1996, we observed a number of cases of streptococcal TSS/necrotizing fasciitis in northeastern Ohio that were caused by GAS serogroup M_3. Invasive M_3 isolates seen in the Akron, Ohio area demonstrated the same DNA banding profile by pulsed-field gel electrophoresis. A survey of GAS recovered from blood and wound specimens from invasive and noninvasive cases during the same period showed that, although this distinct M_3 clone was isolated from approximately 30% of the specimens, most patients did not have invasive disease. These and other observations underscore the role of the host in determining the severity of streptococcal infection.

Case Definition

A working group of clinicians, microbiologists, and epidemiologists established criteria for the differential diagnosis of streptococcal TSS (The Working Group on Severe Streptococcal Infections, Table 8-1). This group defined streptococcal TSS as any GAS infection associated with early onset of shock and organ failure. Because approximately 50% of patients with streptococcal TSS have GAS necrotizing fasciitis, a case definition of streptococcal TSS with GAS necrotizing fasciitis was also included. However, in most series of GAS necrotizing fasciitis, about 50% of cases have been associated with TSS.

GAS Necrotizing Fasciitis: Characteristics and Clinical Manifestations
Epidemiology

During the past decade, numerous reports of GAS necrotizing fasciitis have been published worldwide. In the largest population surveillance study of GAS necrotizing fasciitis, Kaul et al in 1995 reported the incidence as 0.4 cases/100,000 people. Mortality rates have ranged from 20% to 60%. Cases tend to be sporadic. Secondary cases are rare but have been reported among family members with intimate contact and among medical personnel caring for patients. Large outbreaks of GAS necrotizing fasciitis have not occurred, yet identical strains have caused pharyngitis in diverse geographic locations. Therefore, acquisition of the strain is not sufficient to cause GAS necrotizing fasciitis. Thus, a predisposing condition—trauma, chicken pox, surgery, or childbirth—is necessary. In addition, invasive disease may be sporadic because the vast majority of the population has acquired immunity to one or more of the streptococcal virulence factors.

Original reports of GAS necrotizing fasciitis over the past decade emphasized that cases often occurred in young, previously healthy patients. Although GAS necrotizing fasciitis may occur at any age, Kaul et al observed a higher incidence in elderly patients (>65 years) and in patients with underlying disease (ie, diabetes,

8

Table 8-1: Case Definitions of Streptococcal Toxic Shock Syndrome and GAS Necrotizing Fasciitis*

A diagnosis of streptococcal TSS requires:

1. Isolation of group A *Streptococcus* (GAS) from a sterile or nonsterile body site

2. Clinical signs of severity, ie, hypotension

3. Clinical and laboratory abnormalities, ie, two or more of the following:
   - Renal impairment
   - Coagulopathy
   - Liver abnormalities
   - Acute respiratory distress syndrome
   - Extensive tissue necrosis (ie, necrotizing fasciitis)
   - Erythematous rash

Definite Case=Isolation of GAS from a sterile body site *plus* clinical signs of severity and at least two of the clinical and laboratory abnormalities.

Probable Case=Isolation of GAS from a nonsterile body site *plus* clinical signs of severity and at least two of the clinical and laboratory abnormalities.

A definite diagnosis
of GAS necrotizing fasciitis requires:

1. Necrosis of soft tissues with involvement of the fascia

2. Serious systemic disease, including one or more of the following:
   - Death
   - Shock (systolic blood pressure <90 mm Hg)
   - Disseminated intravascular coagulopathy
   - Failure of organ systems, such as respiratory, liver, or renal failure

3. Isolation of GAS from a normally sterile body site

A suspected diagnosis
of GAS necrotizing fasciitis requires:

1. Findings 1 and 2 above *plus* serologic confirmation of GAS infection by a fourfold rise against:
   - Streptolysin O
   - DNAse B

2. Findings 1 and 2 above *plus* histologic confirmation, such as:
   - Gram-positive cocci in a necrotic soft-tissue infection

*Streptococcal TSS is any GAS infection associated with early onset of shock and organ failure. Definitions describing criteria for shock, organ failure, definite cases, and probable cases are included.

Source: Defining the group A streptococcal toxic shock syndrome; rationale and consensus definition. The Working Group on Severe Streptococcal Infections. *JAMA* 1993;269:390-391.

8

alcoholism, chronic cardiac disease, peripheral vascular disease [PVD]).

Transmission characterisics of invasive GAS infection are unclear. The uncommon reports of clustering GAS necrotizing fasciitis cases suggest that transmission may be inefficient. Although strains causing soft-tissue infection do not appear to be easily spread within communities that have acceptable hygiene, patient-to-patient transmission or transmission to health-care personnel has occurred. Pharyngitis caused by GAS is known to be readily spread by direct person-to-person contact, often through droplets of saliva or by respiratory secretions. It is unclear how transmission of GAS occurs from patients with necrotizing fasciitis; however, an investigation of nosocomial pneumonia, fatal cases on a medical ward pointed to asymptomatic or symptomatic pharyngeal carriage of GAS by health-care personnel as possible ways of transmission. This may have significant implications for preventive therapy.

Predisposing Factors

Infection often occurs after penetrating or blunt traumatic injury to the site involved; but it can occur without any preceding noticeable injury. Other predisposing factors include varicella, chronic skin conditions (ie, decubitus/ischemic ulcers, psoriasis), and previous surgery. Our own experience, as well as that of others, suggests that the use of nonsteroidal anti-inflammatory drugs (NSAIDs) is linked to the progression of invasive GAS infections, including necrotizing fasciitis. A review of cases by Stevens et al found that, in several cases, patients' pain was erroneously attributed to phlebitis, muscle strain, bursitis, or arthritis. Many of these patients received NSAIDs without antibiotics, and the disease progressed despite the fact that NSAIDs reduced the signs and symptoms of inflammation. In many cases, GAS necrotizing fasciitis was not established until signs of shock or tissue gangrene were apparent. As indicated by Stevens, a biochemical rationale could support an association with NSAIDs. Although NSAIDs are often used to relieve pain and reduce fever, they also alter granulocyte function. In addition, NSAIDs enhance production of TNF-α, probably by preventing feedback inhibitors by prostaglandin E$_2$. Thus, NSAIDs may predispose a patient to GAS necrotizing fasciitis by inhibiting granulocyte function, augmenting cytokine production, and attenuating the cardinal manifestations of inflammation in a patient with GAS cellulitis.

Clinical Characteristics

The most common primary sites of GAS necrotizing fasciitis are the extremities. Among patients we have seen, the upper extremities has been most commonly involved. However, Kaul et al found the lower extremities as the most common primary site (53% of cases), followed by the upper extremities 29%, trunk 9%, groin/perineum 8%, and face 1%. Necrotizing soft-tissue infection of the lower extremity or the perineum/groin area is often caused by a polymicrobial aerobic/anaerobic infection, which may include GAS. This is important when considering initial empiric antimicrobial therapy. Characteristics of 20 consecutive patients with necrotizing fasciitis reported by Haywood et al in 1999 are listed in Table 8-2.

GAS necrotizing fasciitis usually presents as an erythematous (without sharp margins), swollen, exquisitely tender, and painful area. Severe pain is the most common initial symptom of GAS necrotizing fasciitis. It is often abrupt and usually precedes tenderness or other physical findings. Thus, pain out of proportion to the apparent superficial involvement of the skin is an important clue. Infection often spreads rapidly into the perifascial space. This space is avascular and has only loose areolar tissue. When injury or superficial infections penetrate to this level, necrotizing infection can spread rapidly and more extensively than would be estimated from the superficial evidence of infection.

Table 8-2: Clinical Characteristics of 20 Patients With GAS Necrotizing Fasciitis

Demographics

Age in years, mean (range)	58 (33-89)
Male gender	70%
Underlying condition	55%
Blunt or penetrating trauma	65%
Use of NSAIDs	30%

Clinical Manifestations

Hypotension	85%
Renal impairment	45%
Coagulopathy	55%
Liver dysfunction	25%
Rash	35%
Acute respiratory distress	15%
Bacteremia	60%

Therapy

Intensive care unit therapy	90%
Vasopressors	55%
Antimicrobials	100%
Penicillin	80%
Clindamycin (Cleocin®)	100%
Surgical debridement	95%
Intravenous (IV) immunoglobulin	80%
Mortality	20%

NSAIDs=nonsteroidal anti-inflammatory drugs

Adapted from: Haywood CT, McGeer A, Low DE: Clinical experience with 20 cases of group A *Streptococcus* necrotizing fasciitis and myonecrosis: 1995 to 1997. *Plast Reconstr Surg* 1999;103:1567-1573.

Lymphangitis and lymphadenitis occur infrequently. Diffuse swelling of the involved area is usually followed by bullae filled with clear liquid. These bullous lesions often rapidly become maroon or violaceous (Figures 8-1 and 8-2, see color plate inserts) and are followed by a rapid evolution of frank cutaneous gangrene, and an extension of inflammation along fascial planes. As tissue necrosis progresses, the involved area may no longer be painful because of anesthesia secondary to thrombosis of small blood vessels and destruction of the superficial nerves located in the underlying subcutaneous tissues. Local skin anesthesia may antedate the appearance of skin necrosis. Thus, overlying skin anesthesia provides a clue that the process is necrotizing fasciitis and not a simple cellulitis. In some patients, necrosis progresses less quickly; Kaul et al have described a subset of patients with diabetes and/or peripheral vascular disease (PVD) in whom chronic underlying ischemia may have contributed to soft-tissue necrosis and in whom the progression of necrosis was less rapid. As previously indicated, streptococcal TSS is observed in approximately 50% of patients.

Laboratory Findings

Leukocytosis is usually present in GAS necrotizing fasciitis. As with other necrotizing soft-tissue infections, an elevated serum creatinine phosphokinase (CPK) level is often a clue to the presence of GAS necrotizing fasciitis or myositis. Blood cultures are frequently positive in GAS necrotizing fasciitis. Bacteremia is a predictor of increased mortality; however, bacteremia is not a clinically useful marker because it can only be detected 24 to 48 hours after presentation. Similarly, the presence of GAS bacteremia is not a reliable predictor of GAS necrotizing fasciitis vs cellulitis because bacteremia is also found in association with non-necrotizing cellulitis.

Table 8-3: When to Suspect GAS Necrotizing Fasciitis Rather Than Cellulitis

- Severe pain
- Rapidly spreading swelling and inflammation
- Pain followed by anesthesia
- Bullous formation
- Necrosis (later appearance)
- Toxic shock syndrome (TSS)
- Laboratory-elevated creatinine phosphokinase (CPK)
- Predisposing factors: varicella; use of NSAIDs

NSAIDs=nonsteroidal anti-inflammatory drugs

Diagnosis

Early diagnosis of GAS necrotizing fasciitis is essential for optimal patient outcome. Although the diagnosis of GAS necrotizing fasciitis may be clear-cut at the later stage of disease (extensive necrosis), it is often difficult to differentiate from cellulitis at presentation. This distinction is important because cellulitis can be treated with antimicrobial agents without surgical management, while GAS necrotizing fasciitis requires timely surgical debridement and excision of tissue in addition to the use of antimicrobial agents. Therefore, clinicians should develop increased sensitivity to patients presenting with apparently innocent cellulitis. Clinical characteristics that should direct clinicians to consider GAS necrotizing fasciitis are listed in Table 8-3. Bullae may be observed in cellulitis without fasciitis (Figure 8-3, see color plate insert). The presence of fever with unexplained severe musculoskeletal pain is an important clue to imminent GAS necrotizing fasciitis.

Another indicator of a necrotizing process is the probing of involved tissue with a hemostat through a limited incision that allows easy passage of the instrument along a plane just superficial to the deep fascia. Other conditions that may mimic early manifestations of GAS necrotizing fasciitis include trauma with hematoma (although fever and leukocytosis are usually absent), phlebitis, bursitis, and arthritis. In a recent study of GAS necrotizing fasciitis by Haywood et al, 35% of patients had an initial diagnosis other than GAS necrotizing fasciitis, including sciatica, cellulitis, rash, viral illness, traumatic knee effusion, and bursitis. Each patient who initially presented with a condition thought to be something other than GAS necrotizing fascitis complained of pain out of proportion to that expected by examination, even for those patients who reported previous trauma to the area.

Computed tomography (CT), magnetic resonance imaging (MRI), and routine soft-tissue x-ray may be helpful in demonstrating the involvement of subcutaneous tissue beyond the visibly involved cutaneous abnormality. Radiographic studies should not delay surgical evaluation if necrotizing fasciitis is suspected. Rather, it should serve to expedite and direct surgical intervention. Furthermore, because gas is not present in GAS necrotizing fasciitis (in contrast to that caused by mixed aerobic/anaerobic or clostridial infection), the findings are often nonspecific.

Therapy

The management of GAS necrotizing fasciitis requires early recognition and intervention. Antibiotics, aggressive surgical debridement, and critical care unit support are the mainstays of management. Kaul et al reported that the mortality rate approaches 100% if appropriate surgical intervention is not performed. Although necrotizing cutaneous infections are generally classified based on selected clinical characteristics and etiology (ie, necrotizing fasciitis or *Clostridium* myonecrosis), the initial clinical manifesta-

8

tions are usually not distinctive. Regardless of the etiology, the primary therapy is emergent surgical intervention and appropriate antimicrobial therapy.

Surgical Therapy

The goal of surgery is the removal of all necrotic tissue by urgent radical debridement, maximal preservation of viable skin, and achievement of hemostasis. Amputation may be necessary to remove all nonviable tissue. A second-look procedure is usally necessary within 12 to 24 hours to reculture and further remove all necrotic and infected materials that may have been missed. McHenry et al determined the risk factors of mortality in 65 patients with GAS necrotizing fasciitis. GAS accounted for 53% of monomicrobial infections. An average of 3.3 operative debridements/patient, and amputation in several patients, were required to control the infection (Figures 8-4a and 8-4b, see color plate inserts).

Antimicrobial Therapy

GAS continues to be susceptible to numerous antimicrobials. However, it is usually difficult to determine the specific bacterial etiology (ie, GAS vs another pathogen or mixed aerobic/anaerobic organisms) based on the initial clinical presentation. Empiric antibiotic therapy should be started as soon as GAS is suspected. The antimicrobial agents chosen should have activity against *Streptococcus*, *Staphylococcus*, *Clostridium*, and mixed aerobic/anaerobic organisms, unless GAS is documented. β-Lactam/β-lactamase inhibitors such as ticarcillin/clavulanate (Timentin®) and piperacillin/tazobactam (Zosyn®IV) or a carbapenem (imipenem/cilastatin [Primaxin®] or meropenem [Merrem®, Merrem®IV]) should provide the adequate spectrum. However, it has been shown that penicillin is not effective in the presence of a large inoculum of bacteria (see discussion in Chapter 7). Clindamycin, on the other hand, has shown greater efficacy in experimental fulminant streptococcal infection (see Chapter 7). We therefore recommend initial therapy with a β-lactam/β-lactamase inhibitor combination plus clindamycin until the etiology is known (see Chapter 7, Table 7-3). Tetanus prophylaxis should be considered in patients who are not up to date with their immunizations.

Other Therapeutic Interventions

Because of the high mortality rate associated with GAS necrotizing fasciitis, adjuvant therapies have been considered. Of these, intravenous immunoglobulin (IVIG) appears to be most promising for potentially improving outcome. Early anecdotal reports have also shown beneficial effects for TSS. The mechanism by which IVIG improves outcome in patients with severe invasive GAS infections is not fully understood. However, it has been demonstrated that antibodies against streptococcal superantigens are transferred to patient's plasma after administration. The beneficial effect of IVIG is most likely related to an inhibition of T-cell proliferation and cytokine production induced by streptococcal antigens. On the basis of an observational study, Kaul et al reported a beneficial effect of IVIG for patients with GAS TSS. Twenty-one consecutive patients were treated with IVIG (median dose=2 g/kg) and compared with 32 patients with GAS TSS who did not receive IVIG (historical controls). The proportion of cases with 30-day survival was higher in patients treated with IVIG (67% vs 34%; P=0.02). Furthermore, the authors observed that IVIG therapy enhanced the ability of patient plasma to neutralize bacterial mitogenicity and reduce T-cell production of IL-6 and TNF-α. In an additional study that evaluated 20 patients with GAS necrotizing fasciitis or myonecrosis, Haywood et al reported 16 cases treated with IVIG (>1 mg/kg). The case fatality rate was 19%, which was compared with a case fatality rate of 25% (1 of 4) in patients who did not receive IVIG (not a significant difference). We agree with the authors that the lower fatality rate in this study is noteworthy, suggesting the possible utility of this adjuvant therapy in patients with GAS necrotizing fasciitis. It now appears reasonable to administer IVIG for patients with severe

8

GAS necrotizing fasciitis. However, a concern remains tht a standardized IVIG preparation with known quanities of neutralizing antibody is not available.

HBO is controversial as a therapy for this disease. However, no controlled study has demonstrated the clear efficacy of this therapy for GAS necrotizing fasciitis; furthermore surgery and antimicrobial therapy should not be postponed if HBO is considered.

Prevention

The potential devastation of GAS necrotizing fasciitis, coupled with observations of occasional transmission, has raised the consideration for preventive antimicrobial therapy for people in close contact to cases. Indeed, the paranoia often associated with this infection parallels that observed with cases of acute meningococcal infection. Because of the relatively low incidence of GAS necrotizing fasciitis, it is unlikely that controlled clinical trials will be performed.

Based on several observations of familial and health-care provider transmission, some researchers have recommended two possible strategies: administer preventive treatment to those in contact with secretions, or culture specimens from close contacts and treat those for whom cultures are positive. More recently, the Ontario Ministry of Health has adopted recommendations for preventive therapy of close contacts to GAS TSS. It recommends therapy with cephalexin (or erythromycin if allergic) for 10 days for the following groups in contact with patients with GAS TSS or GAS necrotizing fasciitis, or with patients who died because of invasive GAS:

- All family members (>4 hours contact/day)
- Health-care personnel in close contact with affected patients
- Anyone whose open wound or mucous membranes are splashed with infected tissue

Based on the present state of knowledge, we believe that this is a reasonable approach.

Selected Readings

Barnham M, Holm SE: Serious *Streptococcus pyogenes* disease. *Clin Microbiol Infect* 1997;3:250-260.

Barnham M, Weightman N, Chapman S, et al: Two clusters of invasive *Streptococcus pyogenes* infection in England. *Adv Exp Med Biol* 1997;418:67-69.

Bisno AL, Stevens DL: Streptococcal infections of skin and soft tissues. *N Engl J Med* 1996;334:240-245.

Chaussee M, Liu J, Stevens DL, et al: Genetic and phenotypic diversity among isolates of *Streptococcus pyogenes* from invasive infections. *J Infect Dis* 1996;173:901-908.

Cleary PP, Kaplan EL, Handley JP, et al: Clonal basis for resurgence of serious *Streptococcus pyogenes* disease in the 1980s. *Lancet* 1992;339:518-521.

Defining the group A streptococcal toxic shock syndrome: rationale and consensus definition. The Working Group on Severe Streptococcal Infections. *JAMA* 1993;269:390-391.

DiPersio JR, File TM, Stevens DL, et al: Spread of serious disease-producing M3 clones of group A *Streptococcus* among family members and health care workers. *Clin Infect Dis* 1996;22:490-495.

DiPersio JR, Stevens DL, Beach JA, et al: *Molecular Analysis of Invasive M3 Group A Streptococcus Clones from Akron and Other Geographic Locations.* Miami Beach, FL, American Society for Microbiology, 1997.

Drake DB, Woods JA, Bill TJ, et al: Magnetic resonance imaging in the early diagnosis of group A β streptococcal necrotizing fasciitis: a case report. *J Emerg Med* 1998;16:403-407.

File TM, Tan JS: Group A *Streptococcus* necrotizing fasciitis. *Compr Ther* 2000;26:73-81.

Gamba MA, Martinelli M, Schaad HJ, et al: Familial transmission of a serious disease-producing group A *Streptococcus* clone: case reports and review. *Clin Infect Dis* 1997;24:1118-1121.

Gemmell CG, Peterson PK, Schmeling D, et al: Potentiation of opsonization and phagocytosis of *Streptococcus pyogenes* following growth in the presence of clindamycin. *J Clin Invest* 1981;67:1249-1256.

Giuliano A, Lewis F Jr, Hadley K, et al: Bacteriology of necrotizing fasciitis. *Am J Surg* 1977;134:52-57.

8

Haywood CT, McGeer A, Low DE: Clinical experience with 20 cases of group A *Streptococcus* necrotizing fasciitis and myonecrosis: 1995 to 1997. *Plast Reconstr Surg* 1999;103:1567-1573.

Hoge CW, Schwartz B, Talkington DF, et al: The changing epidemiology of invasive group A streptococcal infections and the emergence of streptococcal toxic shock-like syndrome. The retrospective population based study. *JAMA* 1993;269:384-389.

Kaul R, McGeer A, Low D, et al: Population-based surveillance for group A streptococcal necrotizing fasciitis: clinical features, prognostic indicators, and microbiologic analysis of seventy-seven cases. Ontario Group A Streptococcal Study. *Am J Med* 1997;103:18-24.

Kaul R, McGeer A, Norrby-Teglund A, et al: Intravenous immunoglobulin therapy for streptococcal toxic shock syndrome—a comparative observational study. The Canadian Streptococcal Group. *Clin Infect Dis* 1999;28:800-807.

Kiska DL, Thiede B, Caracciolo J, et al: Invasive group A streptococcal infections in North Carolina: epidemiology, clinical features, and genetic and serotype analysis of causative organisms. *J Infect Dis* 1997;176:992-1000.

McHenry CR, Piotrowski JJ, Petrinick D, et al: Determinants for mortality for necrotizing soft-tissue infections. *Ann Surg* 1995;221:558-565.

Mollick JA, Rich RR: Characterization of a superantigen from a pathogenic strain of *Streptococcus pyogenes*. *Clin Res* 1991;14:2-11.

Ramage L, Green K, Pyskir D, et al: An outbreak of fatal nosocomial infections due to group A *Streptococcus* on a medical ward. *Infect Control Hosp Epidemiol* 1996;17:429-431.

Shupak A, Shoshani O, Goldenberg I, et al: Necrotizing fasciitis: an indication for hyperbaric oxygen therapy? *Surgery* 1995;118:873-878.

Stevens DL, Bryant AE, Hackett SP, et al: Group A streptococcal bacteremia: the role of tumor necrosis factor in shock and organ failure. *J Infect Dis* 1996;173:619-626.

Stevens DL, Tanner MH, Winship J, et al: Severe group A streptococcal infections associated with a toxic shock-like syndrome and scarlet fever toxin A. *N Engl J Med* 1989;321:1-7.

Stevens DL: Could nonsteroidal anti-inflammatory drugs (NSAIDs) enhance the progression of bacterial infections to toxic shock syndrome? *Clin Infect Dis* 1995;21:977-980.

Stevens DL: Invasive group A Streptococcus infections. *Clin Infect Dis* 1992;14:2-11.

Stevens DL, Salmi DB, McIndoo ER, et al: Molecular epidemiology of nga and NAD glycohydrolase/ADP-ribosyltransferase activity among *Streptococcus pyogenes* causing streptococcal toxic shock syndrome. *J Infect Dis* 2000;182:1117-1128.

Stevens DL: Streptococcal toxic-shock syndrome: spectrum of disease, pathogenesis, and new concepts in treatment. *Emerg Infect Dis* 1995;1:69-78.

Swartz MN, Pasternack MS: Cellulitis and subcutaneous tissue infections. In: Mandell GL, Bennett JE, Dolin R, eds: *Principles and Practice of Infectious Diseases*, 6th ed. New York, NY, Churchill Livingstone, 2005, pp 1172-1193.

8

Index

NOTES

NOTES

NOTES

Contemporary Diagnosis and Management of Skin and Soft-Tissue Infections®

Retail $22.50

Ordering Information

Prices (in U.S. dollars)

1 book:	$22.50 each
2-9 books:	$20.25 each
10-99 books:	$18.00 each
> 99 books:	Call 800-860-9544*

How to Order:

1. by telephone: 800-860-9544*
2. by fax: 215-860-9558
3. by Internet: www.HHCbooks.com
4. by mail: Handbooks in Health Care Co.
          3 Terry Drive, Suite 201
          Newtown, PA 18940

Shipping/Handling

Books will be shipped Priority Mail or UPS ground unless otherwise requested.

1-3 books:	$6.00
4-9 books:	$8.00
10-14 books:	$11.00
15-24 books:	$13.00
> 24 books:	Plus shipping
International orders:	Please inquire

*Please call between 9 AM and 5 PM EST Monday through Friday, 800-860-9544.

Pennsylvania residents must add 6% sales tax.

Prices good through September 30, 2008